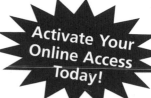

theclinics.com

CLINICS IN
SPORTS MEDICINE

Osteoarthritis

GUEST EDITOR
Eric C. McCarty, MD

CONSULTING EDITOR
Mark D. Miller, MD

January 2005 • Volume 24 • Number 1

SAUNDERS

An Imprint of Elsevier, Inc.
PHILADELPHIA   LONDON   TORONTO   MONTREAL   SYDNEY   TOKYO

W.B. SAUNDERS COMPANY
A Division of Elsevier Inc.

The Curtis Center • Independence Square West • Philadelphia, Pennsylvania 19106

http://www.theclinics.com

CLINICS IN SPORTS MEDICINE   Volume 24, Number 1
January 2005   ISSN 0278-5919
Editor: Debora Dellapena   ISBN 1-4160-2768-8

Clinics in Sports Medicine (ISSN 0278-5919) is published quarterly by W.B. Saunders Company. Corporate and Editorial Offices: The Curtis Center, Independence Square West, Philadelphia, PA 19106-3399. Accounting and Circulation Offices: 6277 Sea Harbor Drive, Orlando, FL 32887-4800. Periodicals postage paid at Orlando, FL 32862, and additional mailing offices. Subscription prices are $180.00 per year (US individuals), $277.00 per year (US institutions), $90.00 per year (US students), $203.00 per year (Canadian individuals), $333.00 per year (Canadian institutions), $118.00 (Canadian students), $235.00 per year (foreign individuals), $333.00 per year (foreign institutions), and $118.00 per year (foreign students). Foreign air speed delivery is included in all *Clinics* subscription prices. All prices are subject to change without notice. POSTMASTER: Send address changes to *Clinics in Sports Medicine*, W.B. Saunders Company, Periodicals Fulfillment, Orlando, FL 32887-4800. **Customer Service: 1-800-654-2452 (US). From outside of the US, call 1-407-345-4000.** E-mail: hhspcs@harcourt.com.

Clinics in Sports Medicine is covered in *Index Medicus, Current Contents/Clinical Medicine, Excerpta Medica,* and *ISI/Biomed.*

Printed in the United States of America.

CONSULTING EDITOR

MARK D. MILLER, MD, Associate Professor, Department of Orthopaedics, Co-Director, Department of Sports Medicine, University of Virginia Health System, Charlottesville, Virginia

GUEST EDITOR

ERIC C. McCARTY, MD, Associate Professor, Chief of Sports Medicine and Shoulder Surgery, Department of Orthopaedics, University of Colorado School of Medicine, Denver, Colorado

CONTRIBUTORS

ANNUNZIATO AMENDOLA, MD, Professor, Department of Orthopaedics and Rehabilitation, University of Iowa Sports Medicine, Iowa City, Iowa

REED L. BARTZ, MD, Assistant Professor, Department of Orthopedics, Division of Sports Medicine and Shoulder Surgery, University of Colorado School of Medicine; Denver Health Medical Center; Denver VA Medical Center; and Team Physician, University of Colorado, University of Denver, Denver, Colorado

ROBERT P. BASHAW, PT, SCS, OCS, ATC, CSCS, Department of Intercollegiate Athletics, Washington State University, Pullman, Washington

ROBERT H. BROPHY, MD, MS, Resident, Orthopedic Surgery, Hospital for Special Surgery, New York, New York

GEORGE T. CALVERT, MD, Department of Orthopaedic Surgery, Washington University School of Medicine, St. Louis, Missouri

PHILLIP E. CLIFFORD, MD, Triangle Orthopaedic Associates, Durham, North Carolina

JEFFREY DIETZ, MD, Northwestern Feinberg School of Medicine, Orthopaedic Surgery, Chicago, Illinois

RALPH A. GAMBARDELLA, MD, Kerlan-Jobe Orthopaedic Clinic, Los Angeles, California

ROBERT T. GORSLINE, MD, The Ohio State University Medical Center, Department of Orthopaedics, Columbus, Ohio

TRYSTAIN JOHNSON, MD, Radiology Resident, PGY-V, Department of Radiology, University of Colorado Health Sciences Center, Denver, Colorado

CHRISTOPHER C. KAEDING, MD, The Ohio State University Medical Center, Department of Orthopaedics, Columbus, Ohio

JASON KOH, MD, Assistant Professor, Department of Orthopaedic Surgery, Northwestern University Medical Center, Chicago, Illinois

LAWRENCE LAUDICINA, MD, Chief Resident, Department of Orthopedics, University of Colorado School of Medicine, Denver, Colorado

WILLIAM J. MALLON, MD, Triangle Orthopaedic Associates, Durham, North Carolina

B.J. MANASTER, MD, PhD, Professor and Vice Chairman, Department of Radiology; Section Chief, Division of Musculoskeletal Radiology; Residency Director, Department of Radiology, University of Colorado Health Sciences Center, Denver, Colorado

ROBERT G. MARX, MD, Assistant Attending Orthopedic Surgeon, Sports Medicine and Shoulder Service; Director, Foster Center for Clinical Outcome Research, Hospital for Special Surgery; Assistant Professor of Orthopedic Surgery, Weill Medical College of Cornell University, New York, New York

ERIC C. McCARTY, MD, Associate Professor, Chief of Sports Medicine and Shoulder Surgery, Department of Orthopaedics, University of Colorado School of Medicine, Denver, Colorado

UDAY NARAHARI, MD, Musculoskeletal Fellow, Department of Radiology, University of Colorado Health Sciences Center, Denver, Colorado

ANDREW D. PEARLE, MD, Fellow, Shoulder and Sports Medicine, Hospital for Special Surgery, New York, New York

ANDREW L. PRUITT, ATC, PA, EdD, Clinical Director, Boulder Center for Sports Medicine, Boulder, Colorado

PAUL K. RITCHIE, MD, MS, University of Colorado School of Medicine, Department of Orthopaedics, CU Sports Medicine and Shoulder Surgery, Boulder, Colorado

SCOTT A. RODEO, MD, Associate Attending Orthopedic Surgeon, Shoulder and Sports Medicine, Hospital for Special Surgery, New York, New York

JASON C. SNIBBE, MD, Fellow, Kerlan-Jobe Orthopaedic Clinic, Los Angeles, California

EDWIN M. TINGSTAD, MD, Department of Orthopaedics and Sports Medicine, University of Washington, Seattle, Washington

RUSSELL F. WARREN, MD, Professor of Orthopedic Surgery, Surgeon-in-Chief Emeritus, Shoulder and Sports Medicine, Hospital for Special Surgery, New York, New York

MICHELLE WOLCOTT, MD, Assistant Professor, Division of Sports Medicine, Department of Orthopaedic Surgery, University of Colorado Health Sciences Center, Denver, Colorado

CONTRIBUTORS

BRIAN R. WOLF, MD, Assistant Professor, Department of Orthopaedics and Rehabilitation, University of Iowa Sports Medicine, Iowa City, Iowa

RICK W. WRIGHT, MD, Department of Orthopaedic Surgery, Washington University School of Medicine, St. Louis, Missouri

CONTRIBUTORS

CONTENTS

> Articular cartilage is a specialized tissue uniquely suited for load distribution with a low-friction articulating surface. Its compressive and tensile properties are determined by its matrix and fluid composition, and are maintained by chondrocytes in the homeostatic joint. Osteoarthritis (OA) is increasingly understood as a family of disorders in which the biomechanical properties of cartilage are altered and ultimately fail as the tissue is degraded by local proteases. Mechanically mediated and cytokine-mediated pathways of cartilage degeneration have been identified in the pathogenesis of OA. Further insight into the basic science of cartilage and OA is necessary to develop diagnostic and treatment strategies for this pervasive disease.

> Since the development of radiography, we have been able to visualize the osseous alterations related to arthritis. These include productive changes, such as osteophyte formation, sclerosis, and buttressing, as well as erosive changes and subchondral cyst formation. However, because cartilage is radiolucent, it is not directly visible by either radiography or computed tomography. With careful attention to technique, both hyaline and fibrocartilage can be visualized by magnetic resonance imaging.

CONTENTS

FORTHCOMING ISSUE

RECENT ISSUES

CLINICS
IN SPORTS
MEDICINE

Clin Sports Med 24 (2005) xiii–xiv

Foreword

Osteoarthritis

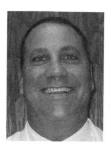

Mark D. Miller, MD
Consulting Editor

How many of our childhood sports heroes are barely able to walk or throw a ball now that they've reached middle age? I've had the privilege of seeing several "aging" former college and professional athletes in my practice and thus submit that the answer to the question is: astoundingly high. Is this simply the price that must be paid for fame and fortune, or can we do something to help? The answer is somewhere in between, and as new technology emerges, we can hopefully do more and more.

Dr. Eric McCarty, Chief of Sports Medicine at the University of Colorado—and a former football player at that school—has accepted the charge of editing this issue of the *Clinics in Sports Medicine*. He has done an outstanding job, and I think you will agree that he has collected some superb contributions from many well-known sports medicine specialists from around the country. This issue covers the gamut—diagnosis, imaging, oral medications/supplements, arthroscopic procedures, osteotomies, joint replacement, and rehabilitation. Although the issue focuses on the most common joints involved (primarily the knee and shoulder), Dr. McCarty has thought to include other joints as well in his final section.

0278-5919/05/$ – see front matter © 2004 Elsevier Inc. All rights reserved.
doi:10.1016/j.csm.2004.08.015
sportsmed.theclinics.com

My hat goes off to Eric for a fine job on this issue. I hope you enjoy it as much as I have. Perhaps we can have some reprieve from the edict that it's tough to get old, because we're all headed there!

Mark D. Miller, MD
Department of Sports Medicine
University of Virginia
McCue Center, 3rd Floor
Emmet St. & Massie Rd.
Charlottesville, VA 22903, USA
E-mail address: mdm3p@virginia.edu

ELSEVIER
SAUNDERS

Clin Sports Med 24 (2005) xv–xvi

CLINICS
IN SPORTS
MEDICINE

Preface

Osteoarthritis

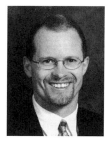

Eric C. McCarty, MD
Guest Editor

The topic of osteoarthritis in sports medicine is a particularly salient one. Athletes of every age, young and old, are faced with the potential of incurring an injury to the articular cartilage. An injury to the articular cartilage can be debilitating and, depending on the severity, may be career-ending. Chronic cartilage wear leading to osteoarthritis is also an important issue that is increasingly being seen, particularly in an active but aging baby-boomer population that enjoys participation in sports.

Articular cartilage injury or wear is most commonly seen in the knee joint, thus most of this issue will be focused on this joint. However, all joints of the body may incur articular cartilage damage and possibly degenerative changes. Therefore, the effects of osteoarthritis on other joints in the body will be discussed as well.

It is interesting that in conversations with many former athletes, particularly football players, there seems to be a high incidence of some type of arthritic changes in their joints. Often there was not an acute injury during participation, yet years later joint discomfort is felt, and radiographic changes are frequently evident upon further investigation. This subject is of particular interest to me, because I have experienced this occurrence of osteoarthritis firsthand. I as well as one of the other authors in this issue both played division I collegiate football in the 1980s, and now, despite no known injury, we both have some early degenerative changes in a unilateral hip joint. We wonder if it was the pounding

0278-5919/05/$ – see front matter © 2004 Elsevier Inc. All rights reserved.
doi:10.1016/j.csm.2004.10.001

sportsmed.theclinics.com

on the artificial turf, the groin strains, or the heavy weight lifting that contributed to these changes. The reality now is that we have to modify our activities. We cannot run or play basketball, but can participate in activities such as biking. What about others in the same boat? How can they avoid further degeneration of their joints? Were previous injuries to their knees or shoulders precursors to osteoarthritis? Now that osteoarthritis is present, what can be done? What roles do joint injections, oral medications, or supplements have? What about bracing or physical therapy? What are the surgical options? All of these topics will be discussed in this issue. Additionally, the basic science of articular cartilage injuries and imaging of cartilage injuries are very nicely outlined. And finally, in the end, the topic of participating in sports after joint replacement is discussed as well as the final topic of the impact of osteoarthritis on a sports career.

The subject of osteoarthritis for this issue of the *Clinics in Sports Medicine* was borne out of the Advanced Team Physician course a couple of years ago. Topics presented to the audience included "Osteoarthritis After Shoulder Instability," "Osteoarthritis After Sports Knee Injuries," and "Can Exercise Cause Osteoarthritis?" The topics were well received and generated much discussion from the audience. It was quite apparent that this was a hot topic with very little information. It was thus with great pleasure that I accepted the invitation of organizing this issue from Consulting Editor Mark Miller.

The contributing authors have all written excellent articles, and I would like to thank them for their work on this difficult subject. The authors represent a wide variety of expertise. Their insight into the problems of athletes with cartilage injuries and osteoarthritis will be helpful to you, the reader, as you deal with the same problems in the athletes and active patients you treat. Although there is some excellent information presented in the articles here, there is still much that has to be learned about osteoarthritis in the athlete. I would hope that this issue of the *Clinics in Sports Medicine* will generate discussions and spur more research of this ever-growing problem.

Eric C. McCarty, MD
Department of Orthopaedics
University of Colorado School of Medicine
311 Mapleton Avenue
Denver, CO 80304, USA
E-mail address: eric.mccarty@uchsc.edu

ELSEVIER
SAUNDERS

Clin Sports Med 24 (2005) 1–12

CLINICS
IN SPORTS
MEDICINE

Basic Science of Articular Cartilage and Osteoarthritis

Andrew D. Pearle, MD*, Russell F. Warren, MD, Scott A. Rodeo, MD

Shoulder and Sports Medicine, Hospital for Special Surgery, 535 East 70th Street, New York, New York 10021, USA

Osteoarthritis (OA) afflicts more than 20 million people in the United States and about 10% of adults over the age of 50 years [1]. It has been demonstrated that 2.0% of women and 1.4% of men per year develop radiographic OA, although only approximately half of these cases lead to symptomatic disease [2]. OA is one of the leading causes of disability and dysfunction in the elderly population [3]; it has been estimated that the total cost for arthritis, including OA, is over 2% of the United States gross domestic product [4].

In end-stage disease, clinical characteristics including various degrees of joint pain, stiffness, dysfunction, and deformity as well as the radiographic manifestations of joint space narrowing, subchondral sclerosis, and osteophyte formation, are easily recognized. However, signs and symptoms in earlier stages, when treatment may alter disease course, are more elusive. Understanding the basic science of cartilage and the changes that occur in OA is imperative to develop novel strategies to diagnose and treat this disorder.

Basic science of cartilage

Functional structure

Hyaline cartilage functions as a low-friction, wear-resistant tissue designed to bear and distribute loads. It is a highly specialized tissue with unique mechanical

* Corresponding author.
E-mail address: adpearlea@hss.edu (A.D. Pearle).

0278-5919/05/$ – see front matter © 2004 Elsevier Inc. All rights reserved.
doi:10.1016/j.csm.2004.08.007

behavior and poor regenerative capacities. Articular cartilage has low metabolic activity; it consists of chondrocytes and a dense extracellular matrix composed primarily of water, collagen, and proteoglycan. Although cells make up only about 5% of the wet weight, chondrocyte metabolism is responsible for the maintenance of a stable and abundant extracellular matrix. The balance between anabolism and catabolism of the matrix is crucial for articular cartilage homeostasis. The mixture of fluid and matrix provides hyaline cartilage with viscoelastic and mechanical properties for efficient load distribution.

Cartilage has an organized layered structure that can be functionally and structurally divided into four zones: the superficial zone, the middle (or transitional) zone, the deep zone, and the zone of calcified cartilage (Fig. 1). The superficial zone is the articulating surface that provides a smooth gliding surface and resists shear. Also known as the tangential zone, this zone makes up approximately 10% to 20% of articular cartilage thickness. It has the highest collagen content of the zones; the collagen fibrils in this zone are densely packed and have a highly ordered alignment parallel to the articular surface [5]. This superficial zone has the lowest compressive modulus and will deform approximately 25 times more than the middle zone. The chondrocytes in this layer, characterized by an elongated appearance histologically, preferentially express proteins that have lubricating and protective functions and secrete relatively little proteoglycan [6]. Among the proteins involved in surface lubrication, superficial zone protein (SZP) has been identified as a functionally important molecule; additionally, the ability to biosynthesize SZP has been used to phenotypically distinguish superficial zone chondrocytes from those in deeper layers [7,8]. The identification of phenotypically distinct chondrocytes in different cartilage zones

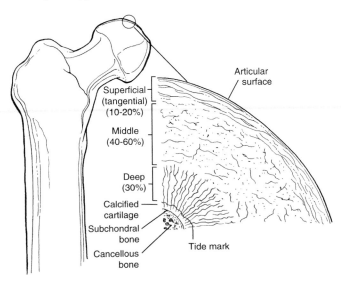

Fig. 1. Stratified structure of cartilage demonstrating zonal arrangement. (*From* Brinker MR, Miller MD. Fundamentals of orthopaedics. Philadelphia: WB Saunders; 1999. p. 9; with permission.)

has generated tissue engineering strategies to recapitulate the zones from chondrocyte subpopulations [9].

The middle zone encompasses 40% to 60% of the articular cartilage volume. This zone has a higher compressive modulus than the superficial zone and a less organized arrangement of the collagen fibers. The collagen fibrils of the middle zone are thicker fibers, are packed loosely, and are aligned obliquely to the surface. Chondrocytes in this layer are more rounded than in the superficial layer. The deep zone makes up 30% of the cartilage and consists of large diameter collagen fibrils oriented perpendicular to the articular surface. This layer contains the highest proteoglycan and lowest water concentration, and has the highest compressive modulus. The chondrocytes are typically arranged in columnar fashion parallel to the collagen fibers and perpendicular to the joint line. The tidemark separates the deep zone from the calcified cartilage, which rests directly on the subchondral bone. The calcified cartilage contains small cells in a chondroid matrix speckled with apatitic salts [5].

Tissue composition and load transmission

The mixture of fluid and extracellular matrix provides the biomechanical and low friction properties of articular cartilage. The major components of the articular cartilage are water, type II collagen, and large aggregating proteogylcans. Other classes of molecules make up a minor, poorly defined, component of cartilage; these include proteins, lipids, phospholipids, and various other minor collagens.

The health and disease of the extracellular matrix is best understood when it is viewed as a biphasic structure. The tissue is composed of a solid phase consisting of collagen and proteogylcans and a fluid phase, which is composed of water and ions. The solid phase has low permeability due largely to a high frictional resistance to fluid flow. This causes a high interstitial fluid pressurization in the fluid phase. This pressurization of the fluid phase contributes more than 90% of the load transmission function of cartilage [10–13]. The low permeability of the solid phase and the resultant high pressurization of the fluid phase establish both the stiffness and the viscoelastic properties of cartilage [4].

The solid component of cartilage is composed primarily of a network of collagen fibrils maintained in a specific spatial arrangement by proteoglycan aggregates. Type II collagen accounts for approximately 10% to 20% of the wet weight of cartilage, and contributes to the shear and tensile properties of the tissue. Like all collagens, type II collagen contains a characteristic triple helix structure. In the solid matrix, the collagen molecules line up in a staggered end-to-end and side-to-side fashion to form fibrils with holes and overlaps. Intra- and intermolecular crosslinking of the collagen fibrils serve to stabilize the matrix.

Proteoglycans resist compression and generate the swelling pressure due to their affinity for water. In articular cartilage, the chief structural proteoglycan is aggregan, which consists of a long protein core with up to 100 chondroitin sulfate and 50 keratan sulfate glycoaminoglycan chains [14]. These aggregan molecules

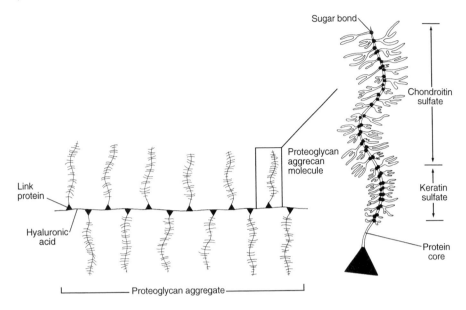

Fig. 2. Diagram of the proteoglycan aggregate and aggrecan molecule. (*From* Brinker MR, Miller MD. Fundamentals of orthopaedics. Philadelphia: WB Saunders; 1999. p. 9; with permission.)

bind via a link protein on the protein core to a hyaluronate molecule. In cartilage, the hyaluronate molecules form a backbone with palisading aggregan molecules; this macromolecular complex is known as the proteoglycan aggregate (Fig. 2). The interaction between the proteoglycan molecules and collagen fibrils creates a fiber-reinforced composite solid matrix. The proteoglycans are entangled and compacted within the collagen interfibrillar space, which helps to maintain a porous-permeable solid matrix and determines the movement of the fluid phase of the matrix.

Water is the most abundant component of articular cartilage, accounting for 65% to 80% of its wet weight [14]. The majority of water is contained within the interstitial intrafibrillar space created by the collagen–proteoglycan solid matrix, held in place by the negative charge on the proteoglycans. Water content is related to the Donnar osmotic pressure generated by the fixed negative charges on the proteoglycans [15]. The fluid phase provides the matrix with its viscoelastic properties—its time dependence, reversible deformability, and ability to dissipate load. Hydraulic pressure provides a significant component of load support of the cartilage, which protects and stress shields the solid phase of the matrix from much of the load burden.

Structure and biochemical changes in osteoarthritis cartilage

Macroscopically, cartilage changes in OA can be seen as softening (chondromalacia), fibrillation, and erosions (ulceration) [16]. Histologic features of

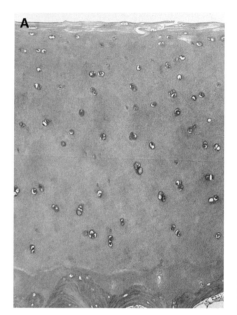 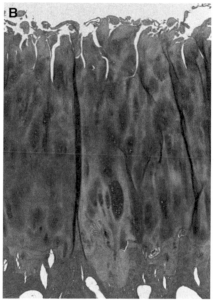

Fig. 3. Histologic section with hematoxylin and eosin staining of articular cartilage in (*A*) healthy adult and (*B*) early OA, demonstrating cartilage clefts, chondrocyte cloning, and chondrocyte necrosis.

cartilage breakdown and failed repair include cartilage clefts, loss of the cartilage layers, cellular necrosis, chondrocyte cloning, and a duplication of the tidemark [17] (Fig. 3). It appears that the superficial zone is affected first in early OA.

The biochemical changes seen in articular cartilage have begun to be elucidated and, increasingly, can be evaluated experimentally and clinically. The OA process is directly linked to the loss of proteoglycan content and composition (Fig. 4). In OA cartilage, a higher percentage of the proteoglycans exist in a nonaggregated form, unbound to hyaluronate. It appears that proteolytic degradation of proteoglycans reduces the chain length of the proteoglycan and inhibits the formation of normal macromolecular complexes [18]. This breakdown of proteoglycan architecture leads to a more permeable solid matrix. Although there is an increase in water content and hypertrophy of the matrix, the increased permeability of the matrix results in a significant diminution of the hydraulic pressure in early OA cartilage [19–21]. This causes a reduction in the compressive stiffness of the tissue, which can be identified clinically as the softening of early chondromalacia (Fig. 5), and can now be quantified with the use of intraoperative biomechanical indentation testing [22–25].

Aberrant proteoglycan synthesis and catabolism produces proteoglycan breakdown products and neoepitopes that may serve as useful serum, synovial fluid, or urine biomarkers to monitor disease activity in OA [26–28]. Recently, dGEMRIC (delayed Gadolinium Enhanced MRI of Cartilage) has been used to directly image the glycosaminoglycan component of cartilage proteoglycans, and may have a role in the clinical assessment of OA [29,30].

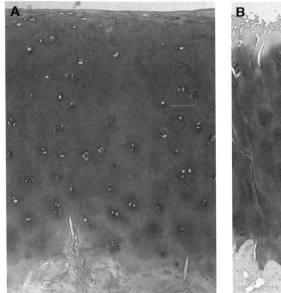
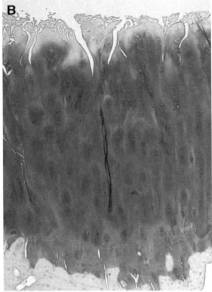

Fig. 4. Proteoglycan loss in OA. Safranin O staining of articular cartilage from (*A*) healthy adult demonstrating staining of proteoglycans in all zones and (*B*) OA cartilage demonstrating diminished staining in superficial region due to loss of proteoglycan content.

There is a rapid loss of proteoglycan content relative to collagen during the progression of OA. However, while collagen content is initially maintained, collagen organization is severely perturbed. This results in a decrease in the tensile stiffness and strength provided by the normal 3D architecture of the collagen interfibrillar network. Changes in collagen orientation in articular cartilage can be visualized by polarized light microscopy [31]. T2 relaxation time is a reproducible MRI parameter that has been shown at high-field microscopy

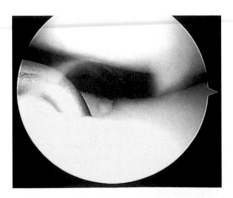

Fig. 5. Chondromalacia seen in early OA. Arthroscopic probing of trochlea from patellofemoral joint demonstrates loss of compressive stiffness in OA.

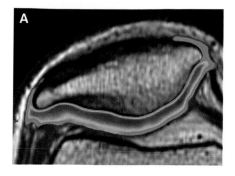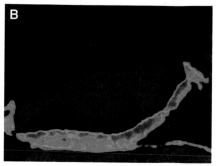

Fig. 6. (*A*) Color-scaled T2 relaxation time map of the patella in an asymptomatic 32-year-old man obtained from a 3 Tesla clinical MR unit demonstrates the normal stratification of collagen architecture on T2, with shorter values (orange) in the radial zone, ranging to the more prolonged values (blue) in the transitional zone. (*B*) Color-scaled T2 relaxation time map of the patella in a symptomatic 52-year-old man demonstrates disorganized collagen architecture reflected by abnormal prolongation of T2 values, particularly in the radial zone of the lateral facet, as well as the central margin of the medial facet. MRI images generously provided by the Hospital for Special Surgery MRI division.

systems to reflect the structure and orientation of the collagen. Specifically, the highly organized radial fibrils of the deep zone demonstrate shorter relaxation times due to enhanced internuclear dipolar relaxations and relative restriction of water motion, compared with the more random organization of collagen in the transitional zone, which demonstrate longer relaxation times [32,33]. Recent work has used these methods at clinically relevant field strengths [34] (Fig. 6).

Effect of osteoarthritis on other joint structures

Although this review focuses on the basic science and effect of OA on articular cartilage, OA involves all structures in the joint. Subchondral bone, synovial fluid, and the synovial membrane are major sites of change in the course of the disease process. In addition to degradation and loss of articular cartilage, OA is characterized by hypertrophic bone changes with osteophyte formation, subchondral bone remodelling, and, in many cases, chronic inflammation of the synovial membrane.

Molecular etiopathology of osteoarthritis

Although OA has classically been conceptualized as a noninflammatory arthrosis due to "wear and tear," it is increasing seen as a mechanically driven but chemically mediated disease process. Mechanical loads, hydrostatic pressures, and soluble mediators from the synovium, synovial fluid, subchondral bone, and cartilage itself ultimately direct the activity of the chondrocytes and the breakdown of cartilage.

The family of proteolytic enzymes responsible for OA cartilage matrix digestion are the matrix metalloproteases (MMPs). Collagenases, particularly collagenase-1 (MMP-1) and collagenase-3 (MMP-13), are thought to be primarily involved in type II collagen degradation in OA [35,36]. Stromelysin-1 (MMP-3) and aggrecanase-1 (ADAMTS-4) have be shown to play a primary role in the degradation of proteoglycans [37,38]. In a homeostatic state, MMP activity in joints is controlled by physiologic activators such as cathepsin B and plasminogen activator/plasmin, and by their inhibitors, the tissue inhibitors of MMPs (TIMPs) [36]. The presence of an imbalance between the amount of TIMPs and MMPs has been demonstrated in the OA tissues. Doxycyline has been shown to inhibit MMP activity, and is currently being investigated as a disease modifying agent in OA [39,40].

Although MMPs appear to be the principle effector molecules responsible to matrix catabolism, it is unclear what directs the relative overexpression of these degradative enzymes in OA. Recent studies have demonstrated that mechanical loading can have effects on chondrocyte viability and matrix breakdown. The deleterious effects of increased mechanical load appear to be most pronounced in the superficial zone [41,42]. A recent study also found that cyclic loading can increase MMP expression and activity in cartilage, although the molecular mechanisms of MMP regulation remain unclear [43].

Although mechanical overload may directly trigger deregulation of MMP expression in chondrocytes, inflammatory cytokines may amplify this response or represent an alternative pathway in OA. There is compelling evidence that inflammatory cytokines such as TNF-α, IL-1β, and IL-6 disrupt cartilage homeostasis and help direct the progressive, MMP-mediated digestion of cartilage matrix in OA [36]. These soluble, inflammatory mediators are secreted by synoviocytes, mononuclear cells in the synovial sublining layer, and by the chondrocytes themselves [44,45]. Proinflammatory cytokines have been shown to modulate chondrocyte metabolism to increase MMP synthesis, inhibit the synthesis of inhibitors of MMP, and inhibit the synthesis of collagen and proteoglycans [36]. It appears that IL-1β is the major cytokine involved in articular cartilage destruction, and that TNF-α drives the inflammatory process [46,47]. IL-6 increases the amount of inflammatory cells in synovial tissue and enhances the effect of IL-1 on MMP synthesis and proteoglycan production. Studies have demonstrated an association between elevated synovial fluid IL-6 levels and effusion, arthroscopic synovitis, and joint degeneration [48–50]. Clinical trials are ongoing investigating the efficacy of IL-1 blockade in OA [51]. The efficacy of TNF-α and IL-6 blockade has been demonstrated in other inflammatory arthritidis but, as yet, have not be investigated in OA [39,52–55]. Other cytokines have been shown to be elevated in OA, but their roles are not well defined.

Interestingly, several studies have demonstrated inflammation, even when measured by systemic markers, may be associated with OA progression. For example, recent work has suggested that C-reactive protein (CRP) may have a relationship with OA disease activity. Although CRP has been used to monitor disease activity in RA, it has traditionally had little use in the assessment of OA.

However, using high-sensitivity CRP (hsCRP), which has a role in monitoring diseases with a low grade inflammatory component, multiple studies have now confirmed that CRP levels are modestly elevated in patients with OA compared with normal controls [56–60]. Of greater clinical significance, in patients with OA, increased CRP levels have been associated with disease progression [60–62] as well as with clinical severity [56]. Recently, it was demonstrated that elevations in CRP are not only present in patients with OA, but may help predict emergent OA [62,63].

Summary

Hyaline cartilage is a highly specialized tissue uniquely designed for load distribution with a smooth, low friction articulating surface. In the homeostatic joint, chondrocyte metabolism maintains a highly structured extracellular matrix that endows cartilage with its biomechanical properties. OA represents a family of disorders characterized by a relentless process in which all components of cartilage are destroyed. It is increasingly clear that this process bridges the biomechanics and biochemistry of cartilage as illustrated by the mechanically mediated and cytokine-mediated pathways involved in the pathogenesis of OA. Further insight into the basic science of cartilage and OA is necessary to develop diagnostic and treatment strategies for this pervasive disease.

References

[1] Felson DT. Epidemiology of hip and knee osteoarthritis. Epidemiol Rev 1988;10:1–28.
[2] Felson DT, Zhang Y, Hannan MT, et al. The incidence and natural history of knee osteoarthritis in the elderly. The Framingham Osteoarthritis Study: the effects of specific medical conditions on the functional limitations of elders in the Framingham Study. Arthritis Rheum 1995;38(10): 1500–5.
[3] Guccione AA, Felson DT, Anderson JJ, et al. The effects of specific medical conditions on the functional limitations of elders in the Framingham Study. Am J Public Health 1994;84(3): 351–8.
[4] Felson DT, Lawrence RC, Dieppe PA, et al. Osteoarthritis: new insights. Part 1: the disease and its risk factors. Ann Intern Med 2000;133(8):635–46.
[5] Mow VC, Proctor CS, Kelly MA. Biomechanics of articular cartilage. In: Nordin M, Frankel VH, editors. Basic biomechanics of the musculoskeletal system. Philadelphia: Lea & Febiger; 1989. p. 31–57.
[6] Wong M, Wuethrich P, Eggli P, Hunziker E. Zone-specific cell biosynthetic activity in mature bovine articular cartilage: a new method using confocal microscopic stereology and quantitative autoradiography. J Orthop Res 1996;14(3):424–32.
[7] Schumacher BL, Hughes CE, Kuettner KE, Caterson B, Aydelotte MB. Immunodetection and partial cDNA sequence of the proteoglycan, superficial zone protein, synthesized by cells lining synovial joints. J Orthop Res 1999;17(1):110–20.
[8] Schumacher BL, Block JA, Schmid TM, Aydelotte MB, Kuettner KE. A novel proteoglycan synthesized and secreted by chondrocytes of the superficial zone of articular cartilage. Arch Biochem Biophys 1994;311(1):144–52.

[9] Klein TJ, Schumacher BL, Schmidt TA, et al. Tissue engineering of stratified articular cartilage from chondrocyte subpopulations. Osteoarthritis Cartilage 2003;11(8):595–602.

[10] Macirowski T, Tepic S, Mann RW. Cartilage stresses in the human hip joint. J Biomech Eng 1994;116(1):10–8.

[11] Ateshian GA, Wang H. Rolling resistance of articular cartilage due to interstitial fluid flow. Proc Inst Mech Eng [H] 1997;211(5):419–24.

[12] Soltz MA, Ateshian GA. Interstitial fluid pressurization during confined compression cyclical loading of articular cartilage. Ann Biomed Eng 2000;28(2):150–9.

[13] Soltz MA, Ateshian GA. Experimental verification and theoretical prediction of cartilage interstitial fluid pressurization at an impermeable contact interface in confined compression. J Biomech 1998;31(10):927–34.

[14] Mankin HJ, Mow VC, Buckwalter JA, Iannotti JP, Ratcliffe A. Articular cartilage structure, composition, and function. In: Buckwalter JA, Einhorn TA, Simon SR, editors. Orthopedic basic science: biology and biomechanics of the musculoskeletal system. Rosemont (IL): American Academy of Orthopaedic Surgeons; 1999. p. 444–70.

[15] Maroudas AI. Balance between swelling pressure and collagen tension in normal and degenerate cartilage. Nature 1976;260(5554):808–9.

[16] Bullough P. The dysfunctional joint. In: Bullough P, editor. Orthopaedic pathology. 4th edition. Philadephia: Mosby; 2004. p. 239–58.

[17] Mankin HJ. The response of articular cartilage to mechanical injury. J Bone Joint Surg Am 1982;64(3):460–6.

[18] Mankin HJ, Mow VC, Buckwalter JA. Articular cartilage repair and osteoarthritis. In: Buckwalter JA, Einhorn TA, Simon SR, editors. Orthopedic basic science: biology and biomechanics of the musculoskeletal system. Rosemont (IL): American Academy of Orthopaedic Surgeons; 1999. p. 472–88.

[19] Akizuki S, Mow VC, Muller F, Pita JC, Howell DS. Tensile properties of human knee joint cartilage. II. Correlations between weight bearing and tissue pathology and the kinetics of swelling. J Orthop Res 1987;5(2):173–86.

[20] Lai WM, Hou JS, Mow VC. A triphasic theory for the swelling and deformation behaviors of articular cartilage. J Biomech Eng 1991;113(3):245–58.

[21] Setton LA, Mow VC, Muller FJ, Pita JC, Howell DS. Mechanical properties of canine articular cartilage are significantly altered following transection of the anterior cruciate ligament. J Orthop Res 1994;12(4):451–63.

[22] Lyyra T, Kiviranta I, Vaatainen U, Helminen HJ, Jurvelin JS. In vivo characterization of in-dentation stiffness of articular cartilage in the normal human knee. J Biomed Mater Res 1999; 48(4):482–7.

[23] Franz T, Hasler EM, Hagg R, Weiler C, Jakob RP, Mainil-Varlet P. In situ compressive stiffness, biochemical composition, and structural integrity of articular cartilage of the human knee joint. Osteoarthritis Cartilage 2001;9(6):582–92.

[24] Bae WC, Temple MM, Amiel D, Coutts RD, Niederauer GG, Sah RL. Indentation testing of human cartilage: sensitivity to articular surface degeneration. Arthritis Rheum 2003;48(12): 3382–94.

[25] Wang H, Strauch RJ, Ateshian GA, Pawluck RJ, Xu L, Rosenwasser MP. Variations of compressive stiffness and thickness of the thumb carpometacarpal joint cartilage with degeneration and age. Orthopaedic Research Society 44th Annual Meeting, New Orleans (LA); March 16–19, 1998.

[26] Chevalier X. Is a biological marker for osteoarthritis within reach. Rev Rheum 1997;64(10): 562–76.

[27] Wollheim FA. Serum markers of articular cartilage damage and repair. Rheum Dis Clin North Am 1999;25(2):417–32.

[28] Lindhorst E, Vail TP, Guilak F, et al. Longitudinal characterization of synovial fluid biomarkers in the canine meniscectomy model of osteoarthritis. J Ortho Res 2000;18(2):269–80.

[29] Bashir A, Gray ML, Hartke J, Burstein D. Nondestructive imaging of human cartilage glycosaminoglycan concentration by MRI. Magn Reson Med 1999;41(5):857–65.

[30] Tiderius CJ, Olsson LE, Leander P, Ekberg O, Dahlberg L. Delayed gadolinium-enhanced MRI of cartilage (dGEMRIC) in early knee osteoarthritis. Magn Reson Med 2003;49(3):488–92.

[31] Wang JH, Jia F, Gilbert TW, Woo SL. Cell orientation determines the alignment of cell-produced collagenous matrix. J Biomech 2003;36(1):97–102.

[32] Nieminen MT, Rieppo J, Toyras J, et al. T2 relaxation reveals spatial collagen architecture in articular cartilage: a comparative quantitative MRI and polarized light microscopic study. Magn Reson Med 2001;46(3):487–93.

[33] Xia Y, Moody JB, Burton-Wurster N, Lust G. Quantitative in situ correlation between microscopic MRI and polarized light microscopy studies of articular cartilage. Osteoarthritis Cartilage 2001;9(5):393–406.

[34] Maier CF, Tan SG, Hariharan H, Potter HG. T2 quantitation of articular cartilage at 1.5 T. J Magn Reson Imaging 2003;17(3):358–64.

[35] Reboul P, Pelletier JP, Tardif G, Cloutier JM, Martel-Pelletier J. The new collagenase, collagenase-3, is expressed and synthesized by human chondrocytes but not by synoviocytes. A role in osteoarthritis. J Clin Invest 1996;97(9):2011–9.

[36] Martel-Pelletier J. Pathophysiology of osteoarthritis. Osteoarthritis Cartilage 2004;12(Suppl A): S31–3.

[37] Lark MW, Bayne EK, Flanagan J, et al. Aggrecan degradation in human cartilage. Evidence for both matrix metalloproteinase and aggrecanase activity in normal, osteoarthritic, and rheumatoid joints. J Clin Invest 1997;100(1):93–106.

[38] Tortorella MD, Pratta M, Liu RQ, et al. Sites of aggrecan cleavage by recombinant human aggrecanase-1 (ADAMTS-4). J Biol Chem 2000;275(24):18566–73.

[39] Choy EH, Isenberg DA, Garrood T, et al. Therapeutic benefit of blocking interleukin-6 activity with an anti-interleukin-6 receptor monoclonal antibody in rheumatoid arthritis: a randomized, double-blind, placebo-controlled, dose-escalation trial. Arthritis Rheum 2002;46(12):3143–50.

[40] Brandt KD, Mazzuca SA, Katz BP, Lane KA. Doxycycline (Doxy) slows the rate of joint space narrowing (JSN) in patients with knee osteoarthritis (OA). Late-breaking abstracts. Program and abstracts of American College of Rheumatology 67th Annual Scientific Meeting, Orlando (FL), October 23–28, 2003.

[41] Chen CT, Bhargava M, Lin PM, Torzilli PA. Time, stress, and location dependent chondrocyte death and collagen damage in cyclically loaded articular cartilage. J Orthop Res 2003;21(5): 888–98.

[42] Lucchinetti E, Adams CS, Horton Jr WE, Torzilli PA. Cartilage viability after repetitive loading: a preliminary report. Osteoarthritis Cartilage 2002;10(1):71–81.

[43] Lin PM, Chen CT, Torzilli PA. Increased stromelysin-1 (MMP-3), proteoglycan degradation (3B3- and 7D4) and collagen damage in cyclically load-injured articular cartilage. Osteoarthritis Cartilage 2004;12(6):485–96.

[44] Sakkas LI, Scanzello C, Johanson N, et al. T cells and T-cell cytokine transcripts in the synovial membrane in patients with osteoarthritis. Clin Diagn Lab Immunol 1998;5(4):430–7.

[45] Moos V, Fickert S, Muller B, Weber U, Sieper J. Immunohistological analysis of cytokine expression in human osteoarthritic and healthy cartilage. J Rheumatol 1999;26(4):870–9.

[46] Caron JP, Fernandes JC, Martel-Pelletier J, et al. Chondroprotective effect of intraarticular injections of interleukin-1 receptor antagonist in experimental osteoarthritis. Suppression of collagenase-1 expression. Arthritis Rheum 1996;39(9):1535–44.

[47] van de Loo FA, Joosten LA, van Lent PL, Arntz OJ, van den Berg WB. Role of interleukin-1, tumor necrosis factor alpha, and interleukin-6 in cartilage proteoglycan metabolism and destruction. Effect of in situ blocking in murine antigen- and zymosan-induced arthritis. Arthritis Rheum 1995;38(2):164–72.

[48] Kaneyama K, Segami N, Nishimura M, Suzuki T, Sato J. Importance of proinflammatory cytokines in synovial fluid from 121 joints with temporomandibular disorders. Br J Oral Maxillofac Surg 2002;40(5):418–23.

[49] Segami N, Miyamaru M, Nishimura M, Suzuki T, Kaneyama K, Murakami K. Does joint effusion on T2 magnetic resonance images reflect synovitis? Part 2. Comparison of concentration

levels of proinflammatory cytokines and total protein in synovial fluid of the temporomandibular joint with internal derangements and osteoarthrosis. Oral Surg Oral Med Oral Pathol Oral Radiol Endod 2002;94(4):515–21.

[50] Nishimura M, Segami N, Kaneyama K, Suzuki T, Miyamaru M. Proinflammatory cytokines and arthroscopic findings of patients with internal derangement and osteoarthritis of the temporomandibular joint. Br J Oral Maxillofac Surg 2002;40(1):68–71.

[51] Dougados M, Nguyen M, Berdah L, Mazieres B, Vignon E, Lequesne M. Evaluation of the structure-modifying effects of diacerein in hip osteoarthritis: ECHODIAH, a three-year, placebo-controlled trial. Evaluation of the Chondromodulating Effect of Diacerein in OA of the Hip. Arthritis Rheum 2001;44(11):2539–47.

[52] Bathon JM, Martin RW, Fleischmann RM, et al. A comparison of etanercept and methotrexate in patients with early rheumatoid arthritis. N Engl J Med 2000;343(22):1586–93.

[53] Genovese MC, Bathon JM, Martin RW, et al. Etanercept versus methotrexate in patients with early rheumatoid arthritis: two-year radiographic and clinical outcomes. Arthritis Rheum 2002; 46(6):1443–50.

[54] Yokota S. Interleukin 6 as a therapeutic target in systemic-onset juvenile idiopathic arthritis. Curr Opin Rheumatol 2003;15(5):581–6.

[55] Iwamoto M, Nara H, Hirata D, Minota S, Nishimoto N, Yoshizaki K. Humanized monoclonal anti-interleukin-6 receptor antibody for treatment of intractable adult-onset Still's disease. Arthritis Rheum 2002;46(12):3388–9.

[56] Wolfe F. The C-reactive protein but not erythrocyte sedimentation rate is associated with clinical severity in patients with osteoarthritis of the knee or hip. J Rheumatol 1997;24(8):1486–8.

[57] Sharif M, Elson CJ, Dieppe PA, Kirwan JR. Elevated serum C-reactive protein levels in osteoarthritis. Br J Rheumatol 1997;36(1):140–1.

[58] Otterness IG, Swindell AC, Zimmerer RO, Poole AR, Ionescu M, Weiner E. An analysis of 14 molecular markers for monitoring osteoarthritis: segregation of the markers into clusters and distinguishing osteoarthritis at baseline. Osteoarthritis Cartilage 2000;8(3):180–5.

[59] Conrozier T, Carlier MC, Mathieu P, et al. Serum levels of YKL-40 and C reactive protein in patients with hip osteoarthritis and healthy subjects: a cross sectional study [in process citation]. Ann Rheum Dis 2000;59(10):828–31.

[60] Conrozier T, Chappuis-Cellier C, Richard M, Mathieu P, Richard S, Vignon E. Increased serum C-reactive protein levels by immunonephelometry in patients with rapidly destructive hip osteoarthritis. Rev Rhum Engl Ed 1998;65(12):759–65.

[61] Spector TD, Hart DJ, Nandra D, et al. Low-level increases in serum C-reactive protein are present in early osteoarthritis of the knee and predict progressive disease. Arthritis Rheum 1997;40(4):723–7.

[62] Sharif M, Shepstone L, Elson CJ, Dieppe PA, Kirwan JR. Increased serum C reactive protein may reflect events that precede radiographic progression in osteoarthritis of the knee. Ann Rheum Dis 2000;59(1):71–4.

[63] Sowers M, Jannausch M, Stein E, Jamadar D, Hochberg M, Lachance L. C-reactive protein as a biomarker of emergent osteoarthritis. Osteoarthritis Cartilage 2002;10(8):595–601.

ELSEVIER
SAUNDERS

Clin Sports Med 24 (2005) 13–37

CLINICS
IN SPORTS
MEDICINE

Imaging of Cartilage in the Athlete

B.J. Manaster, MD, PhD[a],*, Trystain Johnson, MD[b],
Uday Narahari, MD[b]

[a]Department of Radiology, University of Colorado Health Sciences Center, 4200 E. 9th Avenue,
Box A030, Denver, CO 80262, USA
[b]University of Colorado Health Sciences Center, Department of Radiology,
University of Colorado Health Sciences Center, 4200 E. 9th Avenue, Box C277,
Denver, CO 80262, USA

Since the development of radiography, we have been able to visualize the osseous alterations related to arthritis. These include productive changes, such as osteophyte formation, sclerosis, and buttressing, as well as erosive changes and subchondral cyst formation. However, because cartilage is radiolucent, it is not directly visible by either radiography or CT. With careful attention to technique, both hyaline and fibrocartilage can be visualized by MRI.

Imaging of early cartilage damage is important for treatment considerations, because the treatment of focal and limited cartilage damage might be considerably different than more generalized or advanced disease. Focal disease might be treated by osteochondral autografting, autologous chondrocyte implantation, or microfracture techniques. More generalized but not fully advanced cartilage damage might be treated by chondroprotective drugs. The availability of these recent advances in treatment of articular cartilage disorders mandates our having the ability to detect different sites and magnitude of cartilage disease, and requires us to be able to provide postoperative assessment of the integrity of grafts or the efficacy of the surgical or drug treatment.

This article reviews the imaging of hyaline cartilage, including consideration of technique, accuracy of diagnosis, and concepts for future imaging techniques. Because the thickest cartilage in humans is found in the patellofemoral compartment of the knee, most research has been performed at this site; accordingly, this joint will be taken as the prototype for the discussion. The

* Corresponding author.
E-mail address: bj.manaster@uchsc.edu (B.J. Manaster).

sportsmed.theclinics.com

discussion will be generalizable to other joints, although the cartilage is thinner at other sites and therefore more difficult to visualize. Additionally, there are special considerations relating to specific injuries at other joints, and these will be discussed individually.

Radiographic considerations

Radiographs can provide an indirect evaluation of cartilage loss. Weight-bearing images are required. The evaluation is gross; actual measurement of joint space narrowing has been attempted as a simple technique to assess severity of cartilage loss, but has been shown to produce significant false positive and false negative numbers [1]. It should also be remembered that the weight-bearing areas of joints vary with position. The most well-known example of this is found in the knee. Anteroposterior (AP) standing images of the knee may show a very different degree of cartilage narrowing when compared with views obtained in an AP flexed weight-bearing position (Fig. 1). This observation emphasizes the concept that cartilage loss may be nonuniform in a joint, and that standard weight-bearing films may underestimate the amount of damage present.

Magnetic resonance imaging

Magnetic resonance (MR) provides soft tissue contrast that is not available in radiographic imaging, and is a good method for evaluation of articular cartilage. However, care must be taken with choice of MR technique for imaging cartilage. Cartilage is generally thin, and its defects may be subtle. Successful MR imaging of cartilage depends on three major parameters: high image contrast between the tissues of interest, high signal-to-noise ratio of the structures, and the spatial

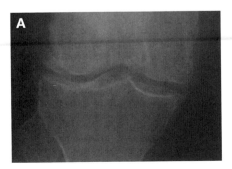 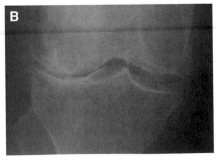

Fig. 1. AP standing (*A*) and AP notch (*B*) weight-bearing views. The AP standing view suggests mild cartilage narrowing, equal in the medial and lateral compartments. The standing notch view demonstrates that there is more significant cartilage narrowing in the posterior lateral compartment. The degree of arthritis is much more significant than would have been presumed based only on the AP standing view. Cartilage thinning is often not uniform; knowledge of this may alter treatment plans.

resolution of the technique. Not all techniques, or MR scanners for that manner, provide equally accurate diagnoses of cartilage damage. Several techniques have been proposed and studied, hoping to optimize the evaluation of cartilage. Some of these are based on intrinsic signal intensity alterations in damaged cartilage. However, thus far, we have found more success with sequences that produce excellent contrast between articular cartilage and adjacent cortex as well as adjacent joint fluid. This contrast, in turn, allows evaluation, on a morphologic basis, of focal defects or more generalized cartilage thinning. Currently used techniques will be discussed in this section.

T1-weighted imaging is frequently used to evaluate osseous abnormalities, because the high signal intensity of fatty marrow contrasts with lesions within the bone. This sequence is not routinely used to evaluate cartilage. Normal articular cartilage is gray on T1, which contrasts with the adjacent low-signal cortex, but

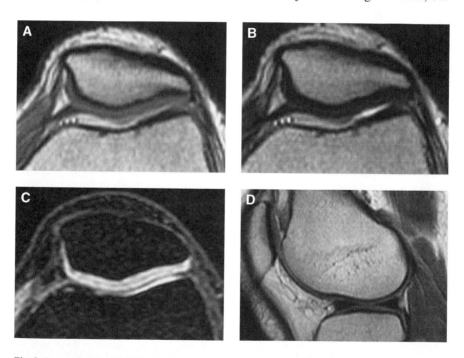

Fig. 2. Proton density (PD) (*A*), T2 (*B*), spoiled gradient echo imaging (SPGR) (*C*) axial, and sagittal PD (*D*) imaging of a normal knee. With PD imaging (*A*), note that there is good contrast between the black cortical bone and the adjacent cartilage; there is also sufficient contrast between the cartilage and adjacent soft tissues that surface defects could, if they were present, be appreciated. With T2 imaging (*B*), there is still good contrast between the cartilage and adjacent soft tissues, as well as the tiny amount of fluid in the joint. However, it is impossible to differentiate between the dark cortical bone and cartilage, making estimation of cartilage width inaccurate. With SPGR imaging (*C*), cartilage is very bright, with a high degree of contrast between both cortex and adjacent soft tissues. This sequence can be valuable for evaluation of cartilage, depending on surface morphology for detecting defects, but is not useful for diagnosing other abnormalities within the joint. The sagittal PD image (*D*) shows how much thinner the cartilage is over the femoral condyle and tibial plateau, as well as the normal focal thinning of the cartilage at the lateral femoral condylar recess.

has suboptimal contrast with any joint fluid, which is also gray. T1-weighted imaging thus is subject to overestimating cartilage thickness in the presence of joint effusion, and to obscuring focal defects.

Conventional spin echo (SE) T2 weighting is also suboptimal for cartilage evaluation. It shows effusions well, but some components of cartilage have relatively short T2 and are not well depicted. Normal cartilage on intermediate weighted imaging (proton density [PD]) is a slightly darker gray than on T1-weighted imaging. The high signal intensity fluid gives an arthrogram-like effect adjacent to the cartilage, but this sequence has been found to be relatively insensitive for detecting articular surface defects [2]. On T2 SE imaging, normal cartilage appears even lower signal than on PD imaging; it can be difficult to differentiate cortex from cartilage, because both cartilage and cortex appear dark. This lack of contrast between cartilage and cortex makes thickness of cartilage difficult to evaluate on conventional spin echo T2 imaging. Finally, conventional SE imaging takes an excessively long time to accomplish, making it more likely that the images will be degraded by motion. This sequence is not required to visualize other structures within the knee, and therefore is not routinely used in evaluating either cartilage or the knee.

Using high-resolution fast spin echo (FSE) intermediate and T2-weighted sequences with long echo trains significantly improves tissue contrast between articular cartilage and either adjacent fluid or cortical bone. This occurs because of inherent magnetization transfer effects caused by the multiple refocusing pulses used in FSE sequences [3]. Magnetization transfer contrast occurs in tissues with high concentrations of macromolecules, such as cartilage. Because of this effect, articular cartilage shows a lower signal intensity gray on FSE than SE sequences, making it more easily distinguishable from joint fluid with intermediate (PD) weighting (Fig. 2). Therefore, cartilage is evaluated for morphologic abnormalities (surface defects or thinning) when using FSE PD sequences (Figs. 3 and 4). It should be noted that, even with FSE, occasionally

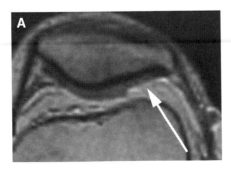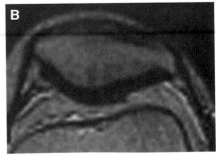

Fig. 3. Proton density (PD) (A) and T2 (B) axial images of the knee. Both images show a large focal defect involving the lateral patellar facet (arrow). Note that there is no effusion outlining the defect, but it is still clearly seen. Note also that the true degree of cartilage thinning is seen on the PD rather than T2 image, because the PD allows distinction between subchondral cortex and cartilage, while the T2 does not.

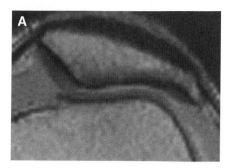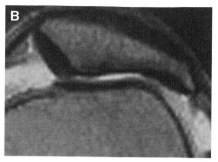

Fig. 4. Proton density (*A*) and T2 (*B*) axial images of the knee. Both images show a large focal defect involving the entire lateral patellar facet. Unlike the example in Fig. 3, there is a small effusion present outlining the defect. The defect and complete absence of cartilage on the lateral facet is seen well on both sequences.

it is still difficult to differentiate cartilage from adjacent effusion (Figs. 5 and 6). With FSE T2 weighting, cartilage appears dark gray (see Fig. 2), and areas of cartilage damage may be seen as focal increase in signal. This is due to the fact that areas of damage have a decreased collagen content; with FSE imaging, there is decreased magnetization transfer effect at the focal abnormality, resulting in focal increase in signal within the cartilage [4]. However, the contrast between cartilage and fluid is generated at the expense of cartilage signal, so small intrasubstance abnormalities may be less well seen [5]. When there is an effusion, T2 FSE imaging shows surface cartilage defects, as does PD FSE imaging (see Figs. 4 and 6). As with spin echo imaging, it is extremely difficult to differentiate the cortex from cartilage because their signal is so similar. Therefore, T2 imaging exaggerates the thickness of cartilage.

Several investigators and practitioners choose to add fat suppression to FSE imaging of joints. This technique increases contrast between fat and nonfat-containing structures, and subjectively may allow an increase in detail in the imaged cartilage (Figs. 5 and 7). Objective differences in accuracy have not been demonstrated (see discussion of MR accuracy, below). FSE PD imaging with fat suppression generally relies on morphologic rather than signal intensity changes for diagnosis. This technique of fat suppression also emphasizes underlying bone marrow edema; marrow edema sometimes is an indicator of overlying cartilage defects [6].

Inversion recovery (STIR) imaging is another method of fat suppression. However, this effect comes at the expense of signal to noise, resulting in resolution that is not sufficient for cartilage evaluation. STIR imaging thus is not a method of choice for cartilage imaging. Similarly, T2* gradient echo imaging was used in early MR imaging of joints, especially to evaluate fibrocartilage (menisci and labra). However, this technique has poor sensitivity for hyaline cartilage because of poor contrast resolution between cartilage and fluid and is not used for cartilage evaluation.

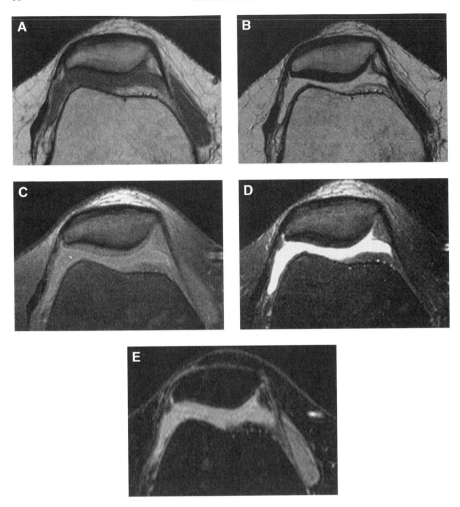

Fig. 5. Normal patellar cartilage in a patient with a moderate effusion. (*A*) A proton density (PD) sequence. In this case, the effusion and cartilage have the same signal intensity, as can occasionally happen, resulting in an inability to evaluate the cartilage for surface defects. (*B*) A T2 sequence, with the effusion outlining the normal cartilage surface morphology. (*C*) A PD sequence with fat saturation; it allows differentiation between the cartilage and effusion. (*D*) A T2 sequence with fat saturation. (*E*) A spoiled gradient echo imaging (SPGR) sequence. In this case, as with the PD sequence, the contrast between the cartilage and effusion is insufficient to differentiate them. This occasionally can happen with these two sequences.

With the knowledge that imaging of cartilage requires high spatial resolution techniques, as well as high contrast resolution to differentiate cartilage from adjacent tissues, 3D spoiled gradient echo imaging (3D SPGR) has been advocated as a method to improve both sensitivity and specificity [2]. With 3D SPGR, the signal in cartilage is uniformly high, with adjacent bone having very low signal (see Fig. 2). The cartilage abnormalities are seen as contour defects

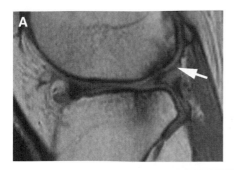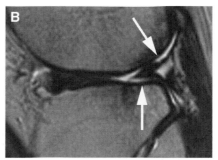

Fig. 6. Proton density (PD) (*A*) and T2 (*B*) sagittal images of the lateral compartment of the patient whose plain radiographs are seen in Fig. 1. As expected by the notch view in Fig. 1, the posterior portion of the lateral compartment should show more severe cartilage damage than the anterior or central portions. However, the PD image (*A*) does not appear to show posterior femoral condylar cartilage thinning (*arrow*). The answer to this apparent contradiction is found on the T2 sequence (*B*), where complete absence of posterior femoral cartilage is demonstrated (*arrow*). The "cartilage" seen on the PD sequence is effusion having isointense signal to cartilage, outlined by the superior fascicle of the meniscus. Note that there is also complete cartilage thinning in the posterior tibial plateau (*second arrow, B*).

rather than signal abnormalities. Contrast between cartilage and adjacent fluid can be problematic [5] (see Fig. 5). It should be noted that these sequences are useful only for evaluating cartilage; there is poor visualization of other intra-articular structures of interest. The 3D SPGR sequences add approximately 6 minutes of imaging time, and require additional image manipulation. Another drawback relates to the "blooming" of intraarticular metal fragments that is often seen with this sequence in patients who have previously had either arthroscopic or open surgery.

In the ensuing discussion of accuracy of these various MR sequences, the reader will see that there is a wide range of reported sensitivities and specificities. This relates to the large variety of parameters that must be specified in these

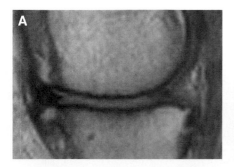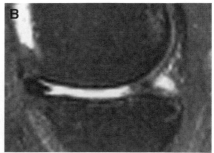

Fig. 7. Sagittal proton density (PD) (*A*) and PD with fat saturation (*B*) showing complete denudation of cartilage on both the femur and tibial plateau. The PD image suggests cartilage damage as well as the posterior horn meniscal tear, but effusion makes it difficult to determine the extent. Adding fat saturation makes the complete diagnosis easier in this case.

sequences. Slice thickness, plane of section, matrix size, and number of articular surfaces, among other choices, contribute to our inability to precisely define the "best" cartilage sequence. Additionally, small sample size in studies with an arthroscopic gold standard contributes to this difficulty. Nonetheless, several clinical studies suggest that there are currently a relatively few sequences to choose from for reliable evaluation of cartilage.

The 3D SPGR sequences are found to be fairly accurate. One study of 114 patients, of whom 48 had arthroscopic correlation, looked at six articular surfaces and found 79 hyaline cartilage defects in 32 patients. The 3D SPGR imaging of all the defects combined showed higher sensitivities than conventional SE imaging, with accuracy of 91%, sensitivity of 86%, and specificity of 97% [7]. The interpretations were most accurate at the thicker patellofemoral compartment, and least in the concave and thinner cartilage of the lateral tibial plateau. Another clinical study (by a subset of the same authors) of 12 patients with arthroscopic correlation showed the 3D SPGR technique to have 93% sensitivity and 94% specificity compared with standard SE (T1, PD, and T2) imaging of 53% sensitivity and 93% specificity [8].

FSE sequences were evaluated in two moderately large clinical studies with arthroscopic correlation. In one FSE PD imaging without fat suppression was used as the standard knee sequence, evaluating 324 cartilage surfaces. By arthroscopy, there were 56 partial thickness cartilage defects and 27 full thickness defects. The imaging showed a sensitivity ranging from 59 to 73% (three reviewers), specificity ranging from 87% to 91%, and accuracy ranging from 80% to 86%. The authors specifically noted that the presence of joint fluid is not necessary to achieve these results, and feel that this routine sequence is comparable to the more time consuming specialized sequences [3]. They believe that routine FSE sequences in the knee are very effective in terms of cost efficiency and the balance of diagnostic needs. Unlike some of the specialized sequences, routine FSE sequences include diagnostic information relating to bone bruises, meniscal injuries, and ligament damage, which are often related to cartilage injury and which should serve as a reminder to look for associated cartilage damage (Figs. 8–10).

This belief that FSE PD imaging balances the needs of diagnosis and time/cost efficiency seems to be substantiated by another group, which evaluated 88 patients, 616 articular surfaces, yielding 248 lesions using FSE PD imaging in three planes. These investigators used the five-point Outerbridge classification system both for MR and arthroscopic interpretation. They found MR sensitivity to be 87%, specificity 94%, accuracy 92%, positive predictive value 85%, and negative predictive value 95% for detection of a chondral lesion [9]. A third group investigated FSE imaging in osteoarthritis of the knee, evaluating grading of chondral lesions. Of 137 joint surfaces graded, the MR and arthroscopic grades were the same in 68%. Grouping the grades improves the correlation: the lesions were judged the same or differing by only one grade in 90%, and the same or differing by either one or two grades in 94%. It was concluded that FSE MR imaging is moderately accurate in grading chondral injuries [10].

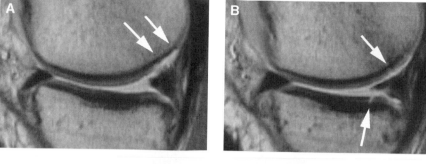

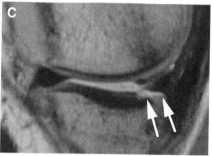

Fig. 8. Sagittal proton density (PD), three sequential images, showing posterior horn medial meniscal tear with adjacent femoral condylar cartilage defect (*arrow, A*), adjacent more focal tibial and femoral condylar defects (*arrows, B*), and adjacent large tibial plateau defect (*arrow, C*). Meniscal tears should stimulate the search for associated cartilage lesions.

Another group of investigators studied the accuracy of chondral imaging when fat saturation is added to T2-weighted FSE sequences. They found, in 130 patients, a sensitivity of 94%, specificity of 99%, and accuracy of 98% [11], and concluded that for many practices routine knee MR sequences were sufficiently accurate for imaging cartilage, and that SPGR sequences are not

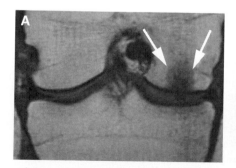

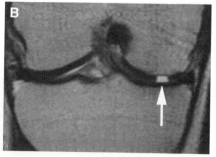

Fig. 9. T1 coronal image demonstrates an osseous abnormality in the medial femoral condyle (*arrows, A*). Such a focal abnormality should suggest that there may be an associated chondral defect. Although the cartilage abnormality is suggested on the T1 image, it is easily seen on the T2 image, taken at the same level (*arrow, B*).

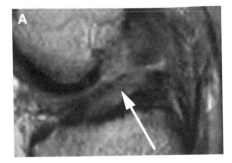 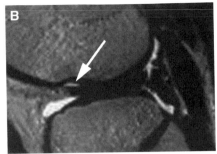

Fig. 10. Cartilage defect associated with anerior cruciate ligament (ACL) rupture. The sagittal proton density (PD) image in (*A*) shows the ruptured ACL (*arrow*). The most frequent bone injury pattern with ACL rupture is bruise of the posterior lateral tibial plateau and bruise or impaction at the lateral femoral recess. The T2 image in (*B*) shows the impacted lateral femoral condylar recess, with fluid filling the cartilage defect (*arrow*).

necessary. They also noted a tendency to "undergrade" chondromalacia by MR imaging in general.

It should be noted that all of these studies were performed with high field strength (1.5 Tesla) MR units. There are many lower field strength units in use today. It is generally felt that these have restricted spatial resolution, poor signal-to-noise ratios, and require longer imaging times such that adequate cartilage imaging cannot be achieved. Additionally, standard fat saturation techniques cannot be used. One group of investigators attempted to separate water and fat with correction of field inhomogeneities on a 0.35 Tesla open magnet to optimize for detecting cartilage defects. They evaluated 19 patients with arthroscopic correlation. Of 59 cartilage abnormalities, 47 were prospectively identified. The reported sensitivity for grade 1 lesions is 50%, for grade 2 lesions is 27%, for grade 3 lesions is 74%, and for grade 4 lesions is 57%. Perhaps more importantly, they reported 22 false positives and 12 false negatives [12].

What, then, is the recommended method for MR imaging of articular cartilage? It seems that, using high field strength magnets and careful imaging, we report reasonable accuracy for detecting morphologic defects in cartilage. However, as yet there is no MR technique sensitive for early or preclinical arthritis, cartilage "softening," or biochemical abnormalities that precede morphologic changes. For detection of morphologic changes, several techniques have proven efficacious. The International Cartilage Repair Society was founded in 1997, and is interested in developing a standardized system for the evaluation of cartilage injury and repair. They established a subcommittee, the Articular Cartilage Imaging Committee, who were charged with assessing clinical imaging techniques and recommending a standardized evaluation system for both native and repaired cartilage. They recommend using FSE imaging with PD either with or without fat saturation, or T2 with or without fat saturation. They alternatively recommend T1-weighted gradient echo imaging; of the two types suggested, the one generally available is the 3D SPGR [13]. Close attention must be paid to the imaging parameters; recommended specifications for specific magnets can be found on the Web site www.cartilage.org. The International Cartilage Repair Society also established a cartilage lesion classification system but it is not yet correlated with the imaging appearance of chondral lesions.

Artifacts and other sources of inaccuracies in magnetic resonance evaluation

The reader may have noticed the "laminar" appearance of the articular cartilage in some of the examples, particularly in the 3D SPGR sequences (see Fig. 2C). When this was first noted, it was speculated that this corresponded to the three zones of cartilage that contained different orientations of collagen [8]. However, this appearance in SPGR imaging is now recognized to be "pseudolaminations," most likely relating to truncation artifact. This artifact can be expected in any region of high-contrast interfaces, appearing as central bands of opposed signal intensity compared with the signal of the object. The artifact is particularly problematic in high-contrast cartilage imaging (especially SPGR). In other regions of the body, such as the brain, truncation artifact can be easily recognized when the structures from which the artifact originates are a different shape than those on which they are imposed. However, this is not the case with cortical bone and its adjacent cartilage; hence, the simulation of laminae within the cartilage [14,15]. A pseudolaminar artifact is also occasionally seen in other sequences, probably caused by truncation artifact. One study demonstrated the artifact in 96% of patellofemoral compartments and 86% of posterior femoral condyles with SPGR imaging, but also in 25% of cases with FSE PD imaging and 21% of cases with FSE T2 imaging [16]. Thus, not all laminar appearances correlate with the histologically observed cartilage zones. However, it is believed that with optimized MR parameters (which are scanner-dependent and not generalizable), that this appearance can be reproduced and shown with in vivo knees and ex vivo femoral heads to correlate well with the location and thickness in normal cartilage [17]. This has not yet been extended to clinically useful information, or a predictor of early osteoarthritis.

There are other artifacts that are especially prominent in SPGR imaging. The signal intensity of normal articular cartilage may not be uniform throughout both the medial and lateral femoral condyles. Furthermore, the posterior femoral condyle shows an ambiguous surface contour in 71% of cases [17] (see Fig. 2D). There is also a linear area of high signal intensity located in the deep zone adjacent to the subchondral bone in the posterior femoral condyle in 93% of cases [17]. Finally, there is susceptibility artifact on SPGR imaging caused by air or metal in 59% of patients who have had prior arthroscopy. This artifact is only faintly seen with use of other sequences [17].

Magic angle artifacts occur at intermediate weighting and reduce with true T2 weighting. They produce an increase in signal in cartilage in regions at a 55 degree angle relative to the main magnetic field [2]. Knowledge of likely locations, as well as the lessening of the artifact with T2 sequences, reduces the likelihood of misdiagnosis.

Normal variants in cartilage thickness, seen on all MR sequences, should not be misinterpreted as focal thinning. In the knee, this occurs at the lateral femoral condylar recess (see Fig. 2D). There is also a normal flattening of the cartilage in the posterior region of the femoral condyle [17].

Magnetic resonance or CT arthrography

Surface morphology of cartilage can be accurately evaluated by MR arthrography or CT arthrography (CTA). A goat model of osteoarthritis emphasized the difficulty of assessing the interface between cartilage surfaces that are in contact with one another, in the absence of interposed fluid [18]. The authors concluded that the optimal choice of MR imaging (with or without arthrography) depends on the anatomy of the joint (whether the cartilage surfaces are closely opposed), likelihood of fluid present, and the type of clinically suspected pathology. An early clinical study comparing conventional MR with MR arthrography (MRA) and CTA in patients with a clinical diagnosis of chondromalacia patella demonstrated a significantly higher diagnostic accuracy of grade 2 and 3 lesions using CTA and MRA; the diagnostic criteria in the arthrographic studies included not only surface morphology, but also imbibation of contrast [19] (Figs. 11–14). A more recent study on 12 cadaver knees compared CTA with routine MR and pathologic examination; for grade 2 or higher cartilage lesions, the two observers scored 85 and 94% sensitivity and 94% specificity for CTA, and 76 and 91% sensitivity and 84% specificity for MR [20]. This suggests that CTA may be even more accurate than MR in evaluating surface chondral lesions.

Multidetector (MD) CTA appears to have a role in studies requiring accurate measurement of cartilage thickness. One group recently reported on measurements of cartilage thickness in 88 sites in the ankles of six cadavers. MR

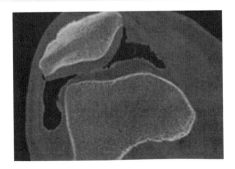

Fig. 11. Double-contrast CT arthrogram of the knee, in the axial plane, allows for accurate measurement of cartilage width.

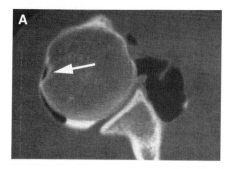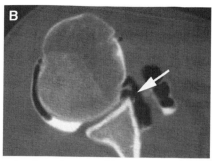

Fig. 12. Double-contrast CT arthrogram of the shoulder in a patient with recurrent dislocation shows a Hill Sachs deformity in the posterolateral humeral head (*A*, *arrow*), but otherwise normal cartilage at this level. At a lower axial cut, a soft tissue Bankart (labral) injury is seen to be associated with a chondral defect (*B*, *arrow*).

measurements were compared with those of double contrast MD CT and the physical dimension. MR consistently overestimated cartilage thickness relative to MD CT and the true measurement [21].

Techniques in development

As indicated above, we currently are able to evaluate cartilage thinning and focal morphologic changes at the cartilage surface with a moderate degree of accuracy. We are also able to evaluate other structural injuries that could hasten cartilage damage (ligament rupture, fibrocartilage tears) with a high degree of accuracy. We are, however, unable to detect early changes within cartilage itself or to predict preclinical arthritis. Because new pharmacologic therapies for osteoarthritis are becoming available that may have modifying effects on early cartilage disease, it would be ideal to be able to detect internal cartilage changes suggesting degeneration, as well as physiologic changes in glycosaminoglycan content or the integrity of the collagen matrix.

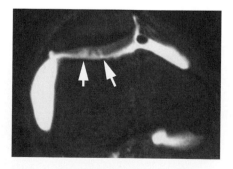

Fig. 13. T1 fat-saturated axial imaging in the knee, postarthrogram. The image shows cartilage fibrillation (*arrows*).

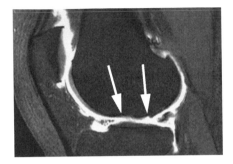

Fig. 14. T1 fat-saturated sagittal imaging in the knee, postarthrogram, shows extensive cartilage irregularity and defects (*arrows*) in this patient who has had several arthroscopic surgeries for meniscal injury.

Techniques are being developed to enhance our ability to detect morphologic changes. These include use of higher field strength magnets to improve spatial resolution, as well as new sequences. One of the latter is termed Driven Equilibrium Fourier Transform, and works to enhance cartilage-to-fluid contrast, with higher cartilage signal than is seen with FSE T2 imaging. Another technique, termed steady-state free precession, and its variants, has higher cartilage signal than standard SE imaging. These techniques require very careful attention to technique and possible artifacts, and are not generally available at this time [5].

Promising areas of physiologic imaging have been reported by Gold et al recently in a review article [5]. These include T2 mapping, whereby the spatial distribution of T2 in the cartilage is mapped, revealing areas of increased or decreased water content, with the latter likely correlating to cartilage damage. Another technique to be considered is diffusion-weighted imaging, which shows the diffusion of water through articular cartilage; in vitro, this appears sensitive to early cartilage degeneration. Sodium MR imaging is being tested, hoping it can depict areas of glycosaminoglycan depletion. Similarly, delayed Gadolinium-enhanced imaging may be used to map the distribution of glycosaminoglycans in cartilage. It is possible that this technique could be helpful for longitudinal evaluation to determine the physiologic state of cartilage repair [22]. It should be noted, of course, that all of these techniques are under development; several require special coils, long imaging times, and are very technique-dependent and difficult in vivo. Their successful development will prove important for the further development and testing of cartilage therapies.

Site-specific considerations

Knee

The patellofemoral joint has the thickest articular cartilage in the body, so is the prototype for discussion and experimentation. The other cartilage surfaces of the knee are routinely evaluated, and there is consensus that the lateral tibial plateau is the most difficult portion to accurately assess, in part because it is thin but also because of its concavity [8,9].

In the skeletally immature patient with an acute knee injury, it has been noted that chondral injuries are more frequently seen than meniscal or anterior cruciate ligament (ACL) tears. The prevalence is noted to be 34% for chondral injury, 23% for meniscal injury, and 24% ACL tears in the child. In the adult, the prevalence of chondral injuries equals that of ACL injury, but meniscal injury prevalence increases to 41% in the acutely injured knee [23]. Therefore, in children with acute knee injury the chondral lesions must be actively sought.

One study showed that the presence of central osteophytes in the knee is an indicator both of severity of the osteoarthritis, but also of focal cartilage defects associated with them. In 200 consecutive patients, there was a 15% prevalence of central osteophytes. These patients also tended to have larger marginal osteophytes, to be older, and to be heavier, all indicating more severe osteo-arthritis. Additionally, 91% of those with central osteophytes had associated full or near-full thickness articular cartilage defects, with the remainder having lower grade defects. The patients with central osteophytes also had more sites of articular defects (average 4.3) than patients with marginal osteophytes alone (2.7 sites of articular defects). Therefore, it seems safe to assume that if an articular osteophyte is present, there will be an associated chondral defect [24].

Hip

Articular cartilage injury is much more difficult to evaluate in the hip than in the knee, due to the fact that the hip is a deep ball-and-socket joint. The head of the femur and acetabulum are closely opposed, and the joint capacity for fluid is small. Additionally, the cartilage is thin. Even with MRA, identifying cartilage lesions in the hip can be difficult [25]. One study showed that staging chondral lesions in the hip proved to be inaccurate in up to 50% of cases using conventional MR; this improved to 92% with MRA [26]. In another study of 42 MR arthrograms, sensitivity was 79% and 50% for the two readers, with specificity 77% and 84%, respectively. These authors noted that 88% of the defects proven at open surgery were located at the anterosuperior part of the acetabulum; the next most common site was posterosuperior [27]. All cases of chondral defects were adjacent to the acetabular labrum and were associated with a labral abnormality (Figs. 15 and 16). It was observed that contrast may be visible between the femoral head and acetabulum only where there is a cartilage defect (Fig. 17). These readers were less sensitive for defects in the postero-inferior portion of the acetabulum and in the femoral head. They noted that false positives usually related to overcalling cartilage abnormalities based on signal rather than contour defects (13% and 9%). They also tended to overcall articular damage adjacent to large osteophytes, again based on signal change rather than contour defects.

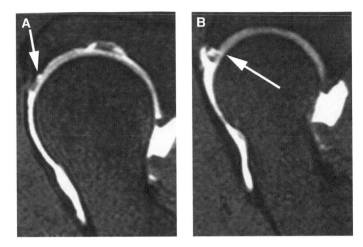

Fig. 15. T1 fat-saturated sagittal images of the hip, postarthrogram. (*A*) A small isolated collection of fluid within the hip joint, indicating an acetabular cartilage lesion (*arrow*). An adjacent sagittal image (*B*) shows the associated labral tear (*arrow*).

Elbow

In the throwing athlete, the elbow is particularly prone to valgus stress injury. This direction of stress results in lateral compression in the joint concurrent with medial distraction. The soft tissue injuries therefore involve the ulnar collateral ligament and flexor tendons. The osseous injury occurs on the capitellum. Because chronic repetitive stress injuries tend to occur on convex surfaces, and because the injury occurs while the elbow is in flexion (as well as valgus), the chondral and osseous injuries occur most frequently at the anterior capitellum (Figs. 18–20). The injury may be a focal chondral defect with or without bone bruise, or may result in an osteochondral defect or osteochondritis dissecans.

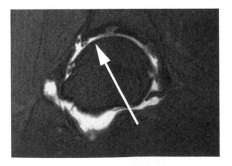

Fig. 16. Magnetic resonance (MR) arthrogram of the hip (T1 fat saturated) in the coronal plane shows a labral tear and associated acetabular cartilage defect (*arrow*).

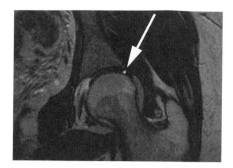

Fig. 17. T2 coronal image of the hip shows a focal collection of fluid between the acetabular and femoral head cartilage (*arrow*), indicating a tiny cartilage defect.

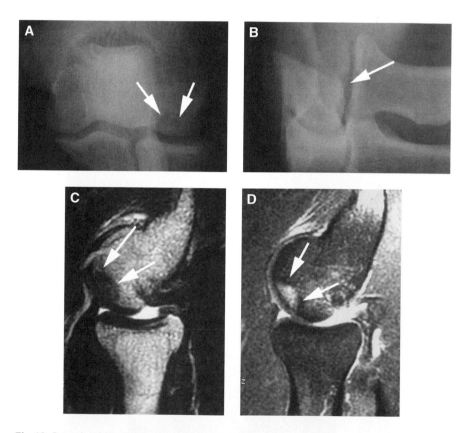

Fig. 18. Osteochondritis dissecans in the capitellum of a college athlete. The AP radiograph (*A*) shows the typical lucency in the capitellum (*arrows*); the defect itself, containing the osseous body, is seen on an angled lateral view (*B, arrow*). The T2 sagittal magnetic resonance (MR) image (*C*) shows no high-signal intensity at the interface (*arrows*); this indicates that the fragment is not loose. The indirect MR arthrogram (*D*, T1 fat saturated, imaged at the same site) shows high signal intensity within the fragment (*arrows*), indicating viability. Note that the overlying cartilage appears intact. This osteochondritis dissecans healed uneventfully.

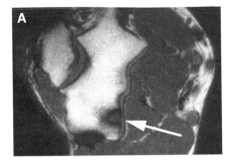
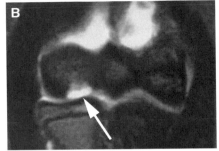

Fig. 19. Capitellar osteochondritis dissecans in a skeletally immature patient. (*A*) Shows the defect on a T1 axial image (*arrow*); the large cartilage defect is shown better on the T2 coronal image (*B*, *arrow*). (Image courtesy of Andrew Sonin, MD.)

Wrist

Cartilage at the wrist is particularly difficult to image. This relates to the thinness of the cartilage, as well as difficulty in positioning the wrist at the isocenter of the magnet. The positioning difficulty may result both in patient motion and in inhomogeneity of fat suppression. In one study, the sensitivity for diagnosing radiocarpal chondral injury ranged from 9% to 62% with several readers. The sensitivity did not improve significantly with indirect MRA or with higher grade of the lesion. The authors concluded that MR is relatively inaccurate for assessment of cartilage at this site [28].

Shoulder

The shoulder is a capacious joint and chondral injury can be seen with moderate sensitivity on routine MR imaging. However, MRA is felt to add accuracy (Figs. 21 and 22). Particular attention should be paid to the cartilage adjacent to glenoid labral injuries. Additionally, the abduction-external rotation position is often helpful in identifying chondral lesions (Fig. 23).

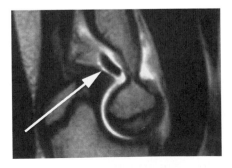

Fig. 20. Loose body from a capitellar osteochondritis dissecans, seen on a sagittal T2 image (*arrow*); the donor site is not included on this section. (Image courtesy of Andrew Sonin, MD.)

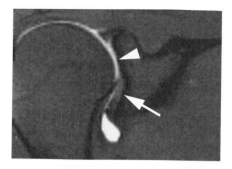

Fig. 21. Magnetic resonance (MR) arthrogram of the shoulder, T1 fat-saturated coronal, showing normal glenoid cartilage at the arrow, but a significant cartilage defect at the arrowhead.

Osteochondritis dissecans

Osteochondritis dissecans (OCD) occurs most frequently in the knee, ankle (either medial or lateral talar dome), and elbow (capitellum). An early MR study showed MR to be 92% sensitive and 90% specific for differentiating stable from unstable lesions [29]. DeSmet et al defined MR criteria for instability of the fragment, including a high signal intensity line at the interface on T2 imaging, fluid passing through the subchondral bone, or a fluid-filled cyst located deep to the lesion [30] (see Fig. 18; Fig. 24). MRA may further improve the evaluation of stability.

OCD of the knee most frequently involves the medial femoral condyle, on its inner aspect (see Fig. 24). However, this location occurs 85% of the time, while the lateral femoral condyle is involved with a frequency of 13%, and the anterior femoral condyle with a frequency of 2%. In a study of lesions in the latter location, it was noted that they generally are found on the anterior aspect of the femoral condyle, close to the midline but usually on the lateral portion [31]. Diagnosis of anterior knee OCD can be delayed, because it may be difficult to

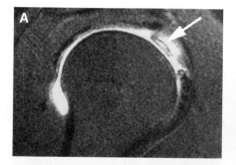
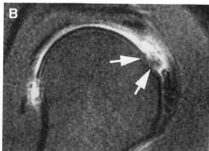

Fig. 22. Sagittal images from a magnetic resonance (MR) arthrogram of the shoulder in a patient who sustained a direct blow to the anterosuperior humeral head (T1 fat saturated). (A) A flattened, abnormal biceps tendon that is imbibing contrast (arrow). The adjacent image (B) shows the osteochondral injury sustained at the same time (arrows).

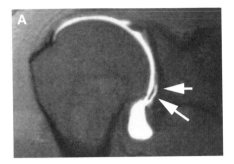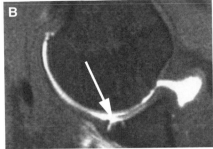

Fig. 23. MR arthrogram of the shoulder, T1 fat-saturated images in a patient with shoulder instability. The coronal image (A) shows the cartilage stripped from the subchondral bone (arrows). The abduction-external rotation image (B) shows the cartilage defect even more obviously (arrow), along with the associated labral tear (GLAD lesion).

see by radiograph; a tangential patello-femoral view is the most valuable for diagnosis (Fig. 25). In this study, the lesion was seen prospectively by radiograph in only 9 of 13 cases, although retrospectively in all. In no cases was there patellofemoral subluxation. Stability was correctly assessed, using the DeSmet criteria, in 100% of the cases, confirmed by arthroscopy.

Postoperative considerations

Therapy for articular cartilage defects is evolving. In some cases, the choice will be to treat the symptoms without treating the cartilage itself. Treatment in these cases includes removal of loose bodies, repair of associated meniscal or ligament damage, removal of osteophytes, and lavage of the joint. With more severe damage, arthroplasty will be chosen.

In less severe cases or in younger patients, treatment is chosen that attempts to restore the articular surface. One such method is subchondral drilling or

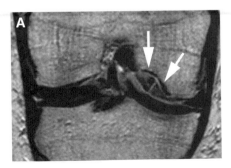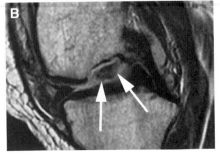

Fig. 24. Osteochondritis dissecans of the knee, in the classic location of the medial femoral condyle. The T2 coronal (A) and sagittal (B) images show the unstable osseous fragment within its donor site (arrows).

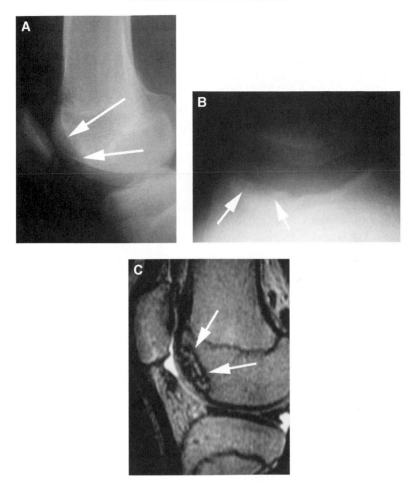

Fig. 25. Osteochondritis dissecans of the anterior lateral femoral condyle. The lateral radiograph (*A*) shows only a hint of lucency, indicating an abnormality (*arrows*). The AP radiograph (not shown) was normal. The axial radiograph (*B*) shows a significant area of osseous irregularity in the anterior lateral femoral condyle (*arrows*). The T2 sagittal magentic resonance (MR) (*C*) shows high signal intensity granulation tissue within the fragment, indicating healing from previous drilling (*arrows*). There is no high signal line at the interface to suggest instability, and the overlying cartilage appears normal.

microfracture. Another is autologous osteochondral transplantation (AOT), which has several synonyms. The donor site for these procedures is usually the knee, and the grafts have been used to treat chondral lesions in the ankle, hip, shoulder, elbow, knee, and even the first metatarsalphalangeal joint. Another type of treatment for chondral defects is autologous chondrocyte implantation, or transplantation. For this procedure, cartilage cells are harvested from the interchondylar notch, cultured, grown ex vivo, then injected at the damaged site underneath a periosteal patch. When this is successful, it produces a tissue that is hyaline cartilage-like [6]. Finally, for large defects, allograft osteochondral transplantation is considered.

Postoperative evaluation by MR is used to examine the degree that the defect is filled, and the integration of the repair with the adjacent tissue (or, alternatively, delamination of the graft). MR can also evaluate the subchondral bone plate and marrow edema. Both the therapy and the postoperative evaluation are evolving fields, and no single methodology has emerged for MR imaging. Observations have been made of a relatively small number of postoperative cases, and suggestions made regarding expected MR appearance. This will no doubt change significantly in the next few years, but the information we currently have will be provided.

In successful postoperative drilling or abrasion, the defect should fill with tissue and develop a smooth surface. The signal intensity of this tissue eventually becomes close to, but not identical to the adjacent cartilage. The repaired tissue is less distinct from the subchondral bone plate than is normal cartilage. Bone marrow edema decreases over time [6].

AOT is evaluated for congruity of the surface. It is notable that the cartilage surface thickness itself may vary, because the cartilage graft generally is thinner at the harvest site than is the adjacent cartilage at the site of the defect. Fibrocartilage-like tissue fills the gaps between graft plugs, and may overly the graft; this tissue appears mildly heterogeneous on T2 imaging and of decreased signal intensity on SPGR [6]. In one study of 21 patients, T2 FSE imaging with fat saturation showed graft protruberance of 1 to 2 mm or else depression of 1 mm, which did not appear to affect short-term outcome [32]. They observed that the graft cartilage usually retains the normal cartilage T1 and T2 signal. The osseous part of the graft develops edema and intense enhancement, with gradual return to normal signal, paralleling the process of graft incorporation [32]. Another group looked at AOT in 55 patients, using MR with and without contrast. Comparing with clinical assessment at 1 year, they concluded that normal findings include bone marrow edema and synovitis, which should decrease with longitudinal follow-up. They also showed partial or complete graft necrosis in six of the 55 cases [33].

Postoperative MR appearance of autologous chondrocyte implantation is dependant on its postoperative stage. Initially, for approximately 6 weeks, it goes through a proliferative stage. This is followed by a transitional stage lasting 7 to 12 weeks, and then a period of remodeling and maturation, where the extracellular matrix reorganizes and becomes fully integrated with the underlying bone. MR correlation is not entirely predictable. However, for the first months the signal intensity of the implanted tissue is heterogeneous but hypointense relative to fluid; it enhances with gadolinium. Once it matures, the defect is filled to the level of adjacent cartilage, restoring the normal contours. The signal intensity remains heterogeneous and hypointense to fluid, with a discernable interface with the adjacent cartilage. If this interface persists with linear fluid-like signal at the junction with bone, it is likely an indication of poor integration of the tissue with the underlying bone. Marrow edema gradually decreases in extent and intensity.

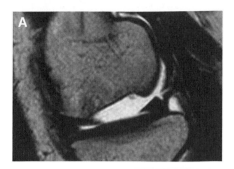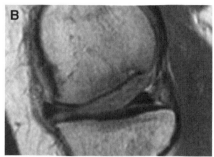

Fig. 26. Large osteochondritis dissecans defect (*A*) in the medial femoral condyle, treated with autologous chondrocyte implantation (*B*). The site of implantation shows good integration of the implanted tissue with the underlying bone, but abnormal hypertrophy of the implanted cartilage.

It is believed that marrow edema persisting beyond 1 year may indicate a problem with the repair [6]. Complications of autologous chondrocyte implantation include hypertrophy or overgrowth of the periosteal cover (Fig. 26), underfilling of the defect, and detatchment or delamination of all or a portion of the patch. Delamination usually occurs within 6 months. If the delaminated patch is displaced, there will be a focal cartilage defect seen on MR; if it remains in situ, diagnosis requires seeing joint fluid in the defect [6].

References

[1] Fife RS, Brandt KD, Braunstein EM. Relationship between arthroscopic evidence of cartilage damage and radiographic evidence of joint space narrowing in early osteoarthritis of the knee. Arthritis Rheum 1991;34:377–82.

[2] Disler D, Recht M, McCauley T. MR Imaging of articular cartilage. Skeletal Radiol 2000; 29:367–77.

[3] Sonin AH, Pensey RA, Mulligan ME, Hatem S. Grading articular cartilage of the knee using fast spin-echo proton density-weighted MR imaging without fat suppression. AJR 2002;179: 1159–66.

[4] Gray ML, Burstein D, Lesperance LM, Gehrke L. Magnetization transfer in cartilage and its constituent macromlecules. Magn Reson Med 1995;34:319–25.

[5] Gold GE, McCauley TR, Gray ML, Disler DG. What's new in cartilage? Radiographics 2003; 23:1227–42.

[6] Recht M, White LM, Winalski CS, Miniaci A, Minas T, Parker RD. MR imaging of cartilage repair procedures. Skeletal Radiol 2003;32:185–200.

[7] Disler D, McCauley T, Kelman C, et al. Fat-suppressed three dimensional spoiled gradient-echo MR imaging of hyaline cartilage defects in the knee: comparison with standard mr imaging and arthroscopy. AJR 1996;167:127–37.

[8] Disler D, McCauley T, Wirth C, Fuchs M. Detection of knee hyaline cartilage defects using fat-suppressed three-dimensional spoiled gradient echo MR imaging. AJR 1995;165:377–82.

[9] Potter HG, Linklater JM, Allen AA, Hannafin JA, Haas SB. Magnetic resonance imaging of articular cartilage in the knee. J Bone Joint Surg 1998;80-A:1276–84.

[10] Broderick LS, Turner DA, Renfrew DL, Schnitzer TJ, Huff JP, Harris C. Severity of articular cartilage abnormality in patients with osteoarthritis: evaluation with fast spin-echo MR vs. arthroscopy. AJR 1994;162:99–103.

[11] Bredella M, Tirman P, Peterfy C, Zarlinga M, Feller J, Bost F, et al. Accuracy of T2-weighted fast spin-echo MR imaging with fat saturation in detecting cartilage defects in the knee. AJR 1999;172:1073–80.

[12] Bredella MA, Losasso C, Moelleken SC, Huegli RW, Genant HK, Tirman PF. Three point dixon chemical-shift imaging for evaluating articular cartilage defects in the knee joint on a low-field strength open magnet. AJR 2001;177:1371–5.

[13] Brittberg M, Winalski CS. Evaluation of cartilage injuries and repair. J Bone Joint Surg 2003; 85-A(Suppl 2):58–68.

[14] Frank LR, Brossman J, Buxton RB, Resnick D. MR imaging turncation artifacts can create a false laminar appearance in cartilage. AJR 1997;168:547–53.

[15] Erickson SJ, Waldschmidt JG, Czervionke LF, Prost RW. Hyaline cartilage: truncation artifact as a cause of trilaminar appearance with fat-suppressed three-dimensional spoiled gradient-recalled sequences. Radiology 1996;201:260–4.

[16] Yoshioka H, Stevens K, Genovese M, Dillingham M, Lang P. Articular cartilage of the knee: normal patterns at MR imaging that mimic disease in healthy subjects and patients with osteoarthritis. Radiology 2004;231:31–8.

[17] Chalkias S, Pozzi-Mucelli R, Pozzi-Mucelli M, Frezza F, Longo R. Hyaline articular cartilage: relaxation times, pulse-sequence parameters, and MR appearance at 1.5 T. Eur Radiol 1994;4: 353–9.

[18] Ho C, Cervilla V, Kjellin I, Haghigi P, Amiel D, Trudell D, et al. Magnetic resonance imaging in assessing cartilage changes in experimental osteoarthrosis of the knee. Invest Radiol 1992; 27:84–90.

[19] Gagliardi J, Chung E, Chadnani V, Kesling K, Christenson K, Null R, et al. Detection and staging of chondromalacia patellae: relative efficacies of conventional MR imaging, MR arthrography, and CT arthrography. AJR 1994;163:629–36.

[20] VandeBerg BC, Lecouvet FE, Poilvache P, Jamart J, Materne R, Lengele B, et al. Assessment of knee cartilage in cadavers with dual-detector spiral CT arthrography and MR imaging. Radiology 2002;222:430–6.

[21] El-Khoury GY, Alliman K, Lundberg HJ, Rudert MJ, Brown TD, Saltzman CL. Double contrast MD CT-arthrography is superior to MRI in assessing cartilage thickness in the ankle. Chicago (IL): RSNA Scientific Paper; 2003.

[22] Williams A, Gillis A, McKenzie C, Po B, Sharma L, Micheli L, et al. Glycosaminoglycan distribution in cartilage as determined by delayed gadolinium-enhanced MRI of cartilage (dGEMRIC). Potential clinical application. AJR 2004;182:167–72.

[23] Deppen RS, Connolly SA, Bencardino JT, Jaramillo D. Acute injury to the articular cartilage and subchondral bone: a common but unrecognized lesion in the immature knee. AJR 2004;182: 111–7.

[24] McCauley TR, Kornaat PR, Jee WH. Central osteophytes in the knee: prevalence and association with cartilage defects on MR imaging. AJR 2001;176:359–64.

[25] Kramer J, Stighbaur R, Engel A, Drayer L, Imnof H. MR imaging contrast arthrography in osteochondritis dissecans. J Comput Assist Tomogr 1992;16:254–60.

[26] Bencardino J, Palmer W. Imaging of hip disorders in athletes. Radiol Clin North Am 2002; 40:267–87.

[27] Schmid M, Notzli H, Zanette M, Wyss T, Hodler J. Cartilage lesions in the hip: diagnostic effectiveness of MR arthrography. Radiology 2003;226:382–6.

[28] Harms AH, Moore AE, Schweitzer ME, Morrison WB, Deely D, Culp RW, et al. MRI in the diagnosis of cartilage injury in the wrist. AJR 2004;182:1267–70.

[29] Mesgarzadeh M, Sapega A, Bonakdarpour A, et al. Osteochondritis dissecans: analysis of mechanical stability with radiography, scintigraphy, and MR imaging. Radiology 1987;165: 775–80.

[30] DeSmet AA, Fisher DR, Graf BK, Lange RH. Osteochondritis dissecans of the knee: value of MR imaging in determining lesion stability and the presence of articular cartilage defects. AJR 1990;155:549–53.

[31] Boutin RD, Januario JA, Newberg AH, Gundry CR, Newman JS. MR imaging features of osteochondritis dissecans of the femoral sulcus. AJR 2003;180:641–5.

[32] Sanders TG, Mentzer KD, Miller MD, Morrison WB, Campbell SE, Penrod BJ. Autogenous osteochondral "plug" transfer for the treatment of focal chondral defects: postoperative MR appearance with clinical correlation. Skeletal Radiol 2001;30:570–8.

[33] Link TM, Mischung J, Woertler K, Burkart A, Imhoff AB, Rummeny EF. Normal and pathological MR findings in osteochondral autografts in the longitudinal follow-up. Chicago (IL): RSNA Scientific Paper; 2003.

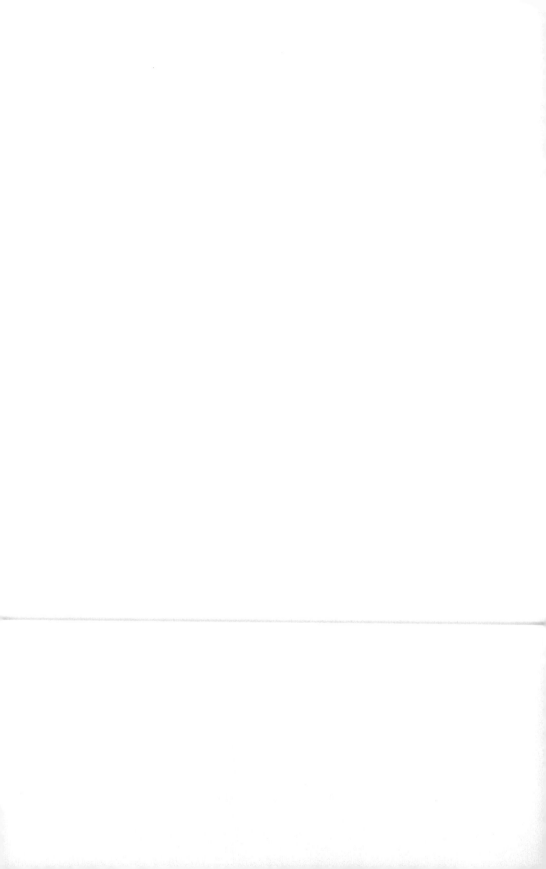

ELSEVIER
SAUNDERS

Clin Sports Med 24 (2005) 39–45

CLINICS
IN SPORTS
MEDICINE

Osteoarthritis after Sports Knee Injuries

Reed L. Bartz, MD*, Lawrence Laudicina, MD

CU Sports Medicine, 311 Mapleton Avenue, Boulder, CO 80304, USA

Posttraumatic osteoarthritis after a sports injury to the knee (anterior cruciate ligament (ACL), posterior cruciate ligament (PCL), meniscus, articular cartilage) is a common occurrence. Although little is known about the natural history of knee arthrosis following a sports injury to the knee, recent advances in orthopedic knowledge concerning the principle of tissue homeostasis has lead to a greater understanding of the pathophysiology of posttraumatic arthrosis.

Dye has introduced the tissue homeostasis theory, a dynamic biologic model of living musculoskeletal systems, which maintains that he knee functions as a living biologic transmission that acts to accept and redirect biomechanical loads while maintaining tissue homeostasis [1–3].

The envelope of function theory represents the capacity of the knee to accept, transmit, and dissipate biomechanical loads [3]. The envelope of function theory combines the concepts of load transference and tissue homeostasis to represent the functional capacity of the knee before and after injury. The envelope of function defines a range of safe loading compatible or induction of tissue homeostasis. Within the envelope of function, the knee joint can maintain tissue homeostasis and function normally indefinitely. The upper limit of the envelope represents a load threshold between loads compatible with tissue homeostasis and loads that induce a biologic cascade of trauma-induced inflammation and repair [4]. Loading outside of this threshold induces a loss of tissue homeostasis.

---

* Corresponding author.
E-mail address: Reed.bartz@uchsc.edu (R.L. Bartz).

0278-5919/05/$ – see front matter © 2004 Elsevier Inc. All rights reserved.
doi:10.1016/j.csm.2004.08.006   *sportsmed.theclinics.com*

Anterior cruciate ligament

Although it is commonly accepted that an isolated injury to the ACL can have a drastic effect on an athlete's ability to perform athletic activities, there is less of a consensus on the long-term consequences of isolated ACL tears and the effectiveness of ACL reconstruction on preventing long-term sequelae after isolated injury. Several authors have shown that in the unreconstructed ACL-deficient knee, arthritic changes in the knee increase with time [5–7]; however, others have found a higher incidence of knee arthrosis in ACL reconstructed knees compared with ACL-deficient knees treated nonoperatively [8–10].

With new understanding of the complex interrelationships between the structural and biologic interactions of the knee joint, evidence suggests that simply reconstructing the structural abnormality in the ACL deficient knee is not sufficient to restore normal physiologic knee function and prevent late degenerative changes [4]. In prospective outcomes studies, Daniel, Fithian and colleagues reported the concerning finding that ACL reconstruction did not prevent the onset of early degenerative changes in the knee [8–10]. At an average of 10 years after injury, reconstructive knees showed great degenerative changes on plain film radiograph that the ACL-deficient knees treated nonoperatively [9].

An important factor determining the risk of osteoarthritis after an injury to the ACL seems to be whether the tear is complete or incomplete. Maletius and Messner evaluated 56 patients who underwent surgery for complete ACL ruptures. At 20-year follow-up, weight-bearing radiographs revealed that 84% of those patients had mild to moderate osteoarthrosis [11]. A higher rate of radiographic osteoarthrosis after complete versus partial tears of the ACL may be attributed to more violent initial trauma [12], or a higher degree of associated injuries [11].

Although studies have shown that although the majority of patients with ACL-deficient knees will develop radiographically detectable degenerative changes, data also supports the thought that the natural history of the progression of degenerative joint disease after isolated injury to the ACL is variable. Studies of nonoperatively treated ACL ruptures with follow-up ranging from 2 to 10 years have detected degenerative changes in 13% to 65% of patients [12–14].

In a prospective study with a 6- to 11-year follow-up, O'Neill found degenerative changes in 11.6% of operatively treated ACL-deficient knees [15]. There was no significant difference in the incidence of postoperative degenerative changes in knees reconstructed with a double-stranded Semitendinosus-gracilis graft with a two-incision technique, a patella tendon autograft with a two-incision technique, or a patella tendon graft with single-incision endoscopic technique. In a retrospective study with 5- to 9-year follow-up, Jarvela showed no significant difference in the rate of osteoarthrosis between ACL reconstructed knees with and without accompanying injuries [16]. Otto reported radiographic assessment 5 years after ACL reconstruction in 68 patients. Twenty-four percent had radiographic changes consistent with osteoarthrosis, which was more common in patients with chronic ACL-deficient knees [17].

Posterior cruciate ligament tears

The natural history and treatment options for a PCL-injured knee continue to be debated and delineated. PCL injuries may not be benign in the long term. Chronic PCL tears demonstrate variable progression of articular degeneration and late arthrosis. Prognostic factors, such as combined injuries, continue to be defined help predict long-term outcome as well as appropriate treatment.

Posterior tibial translation secondary to PCL deficiency results in anteriorly shifted tibiofemoral contact and increased posterior lateral corner stress during knee loading. Anteriorly shifted tibiofemoral contact unloads the posterior horn of the medial meniscus. This prevents the meniscus from distributing the load, and leads to abnormal stress and wear on the anterior–medial tibiofemoral articular surface with in vitro study [18]. Biomechanical analysis of joint contact forces in the posterior cruciate-deficient knee reveal significant increase in contact pressure on the medial compartment in cadaveric ligament sectioning studies [19]. These findings appear consistent with some clinical observations.

Fowler studied isolated nonoperatively treated PCL injuries in 13 athletes over a 2.6-year period. Although all had good subjective results, only 3 of the 13 achieved good objective results in the short term [20].

However, Clancy et al noted 71% of patients at 2 to 4 years and 90% of patients over 4 years postinjury demonstrated articular injury of the medial femoral at the time of reconstruction for chronic injury. Additionally, only 31% of patients demonstrated preoperative radiographic findings of femoral articular degeneration [21].

Dejour et al studied 36 patients with PCL injuries, 15 of whom had combined posterior–lateral or posterior–medial instability. Persistent pain and chronic effusions were noted in 89% and 50%, respectively, at 15 years postinjury. All knees progressed to degenerative arthrosis after an average of 25 years post-injury [22].

Torg et al evaluated the clinical course of the PCL-deficient knee in 43 patients. Fourteen of these patients demonstrated unidirectional posterior instability and 29 combined injuries. Functional outcome was best predicted by the instability type. Combined instabilities were more likely to result in a decreased functional result, as were associated articular injury, meniscus damage, quadriceps weakness, or degenerative change. PCL injuries without associated intra-articular injury or multidirectional instability were more likely to remain symptom free. Notably, radiographic medial compartment changes were apparent in 60% of patients with isolated injuries [23].

Shelbourne et al prospectively studied the natural history of acute isolated nonoperatively treated PCL injuries in 133 patients. They found a trend, although not statistically significant, toward medial joint degenerative change unrelated to residual laxity. Posterior laxity did not increase over time, and grade of residual laxity was not related to subjective scores or objective knee function. In their study, regardless of laxity, on half of patients returned to prior level of sport, one third returned but at a lower level, and one sixth were unable to return [24].

Although nonoperative treatment appears to provide good results in the short term, normal knee kinematics are disrupted, and not all nonoperatively treated knees do well. Additionally, operative and nonoperative management have each provided good short-term results, and prospective randomized studies of patients with similar injury patterns as well as long-term evaluations are required [25].

Meniscus tears

Initially thought to be a functionless, vestigial remnant of a leg muscle, the meniscus is now known as an integral player in the complex biomechanics of the normal knee. Although our literature search revealed no truly prospective long-term studies investigating the association of untreated meniscus tears and degenerative joint disease of the knee, an association between radiographic findings of degenerative disease in patients who undergo menisectomy has been clearly noted since first described by Fairbanks [26].

Several biomechanical studies have demonstrated alterations in the load-distribution patterns of the medial and lateral compartments of the knee after menisectomy. Kettelkamp showed that removal of the medial meniscus caused a 50% to 70% reduction in the medial femoral condyle contact area and a 100% increase in contact stress in the medial compartment [27]. Total lateral menisectomy has been shown to result in 40% to 50% decrease in contact area and a 200% to 300% increase in contact stress in the lateral compartment.

Scheller evaluated the results of 75 patients who underwent arthroscopic partial lateral menisectomy for isolated lateral meniscus tears. Of 58 patients who underwent radiographic analysis 5 to 15 years after surgery, 78% had one or more Fairbanks changes while 84% showed radiographic deterioration of the treated joint. Nevertheless, although the authors concluded that radiographic deterioration occurred with time after partial lateral menisectomy, there was no significant relationship between radiographic deterioration and subjective symptoms or functional outcome [28]. Schimmer reported results after partial menisectomy in 119 patients. The results of 78% of the treated patients were excellent or good at 12 years after surgery. The factor with the greatest impact on outcome was injury to the articular cartilage. The concomitant articular cartilage injuries, which received no treatment at the time of meniscal debridement, became increasingly symptomatic over time [29].

Articular cartilage injury

The natural history of acute osteochondral or chondral injury to the knee continues to be an often debated and controversial subject. Little is known about the natural history of acute chondral lesions of the knee or their link to future knee symptoms or arthritis. Our literature revealed no prospective trial investigating the incidence of osteoarthritis in the long- or short-term associated with chondral injury. Although several authors contend that the presences of an acute chondral injury, seen on magnetic resonance imaging as a "bone bruise," may be a risk factor for future degenerative changes in the knee [30,31], others have found no significant difference in the distribution of IKDC radiographic findings in patients with and without chondral lesions who underwent ACL reconstruction [32]. It is not known at what point articular cartilage injury becomes irreversible and the chondrocytes lose their potential to maintain a balance between matrix synthesis and degradation.

Johnson sought to describe the acute pathologic appearance of the articular cartilage overlying geographic bone bruises found on MRI in patients with ACL tears [33]. Histologic evaluation of the articular cartilage overlying bone bruises revealed chondrocyte degeneration and loss of proteoglycan. Osteocyte necrosis and empty lacunae were noted in the subchondral bone. The authors concluded that a geographic bone bruise noted on magnetic resonance imaging indicated substantial damage to articular cartilage homeostasis.

Faber described 6 year follow-up clinical and magnetic resonance imaging sequelae of occult osteochondral lesions of the knee in a group of patients who had undergone ACL reconstruction [34]. In his study, 15 or 23 patients had persistent subchondral marrow changes on follow-up magnetic resonance imaging that corresponded to the index osteochondral lesion found at the time of surgery. Significant clinical differences were not detected between patients in whom magnetic resonance imaging showed no lesions and in patients in whom magnetic resonance imaging showed subchondral or cartilage injury.

Shelbourne sought to determine if isolated, untreated chondral defects noted at the time of ACL reconstruction had an effect on radiographic, subjective, or objective results of surgery [32]. At a mean of 6.2 years postoperatively, the results of objective evaluation were significantly higher for patients without a chondral lesion compared with patients with a chondral lesion. Patients with Outerbridge grade 3 or 4 articular cartilage defects observed at the time of arthroscopy had significantly lower subjective scores than patients without a chondral defect. There was no significant correlation between defect size and subjective scores. There was no significant difference in the distribution of radiographic findings between patients with and without chondral lesions.

Summary

Recent advances in the knowledge of tissue homeostasis, including the tissue homeostasis theory and the envelope of function theory as proposed by Dye, have greatly increased our knowledge of the pathophysiology of osteoarthrosis after sports knee injuries. The development of these two theories has not only advanced our understanding of the treatment and prevention of osteoarthrosis after acute injuries to the knee, but has also given us guidance as to directions for future research.

References

[1] Dye SF, Chew MH, McBride JT, Sostre G. Restoration of osseous homeostasis of the knee following meniscus surgery. Ortho Transact 1992;16:725–6.

[2] Dye SF, Chew MH. Restoration of osseous homeostasis after anterior cruciate ligament reconstruction. Am J Sports Med 1993;21:748–50.

[3] Dye SF. The knee as a biologic transmission with an envelope of function. Clin Orthop 1996; 325:10–8.

[4] Dye SF, Wojtys EM, Fu FH, Fithian DC, Gillquist J. Factors contributing to function of the knee after injury or reconstruction of the anterior cruciate ligament. J Bone Joint Surg 1998; 80A(9):1380–93.

[5] Hawkins RJ, Misamore GW, Merritt TR. Followup of the acute nonoperated isolated anterior cruciate ligament tear. Am J Sports Med 1986;14:205–10.

[6] Fowler PJ, Regan WD. The patient with symptomatic chronic anterior cruciate ligament insufficiency. Results of minimal arthroscopic surgery and rehabilitation. Am J Sports Med 1987;5:321–5.

[7] Buss DD, Min R, Skyhar M, Galinat B, Warren RF, Wickiewicz TL. Nonoperative treatment of acute anterior cruciate ligament injuries in a selected group of patients. Am J Sports Med 1995;23:160–5.

[8] Daniel DM, Stone ML, Dobson BE, Fithian DC, Rossman DJ, Kaufman KR. Fate of the ACL injured patient. A prospective outcome study. Am J Sports Med 1994;22:633–44.

[9] Daniel DM, Fithian DC, Stone ML, Dobson BE, Luetzow WF, Kaufman KR. A ten year prospective outcome study of the ACL-injured patient. Orthop Trans 1996;20:700–1.

[10] Fithian DC. The fate of the anterior cruciate ligament injured patient: long-term follow-up: the San Diego experience. Presented at the Annual Meeting of the American Academy of Orthopedic Surgeons, San Francisco (CA), February 14, 1997.

[11] Maletius W, Messner K. Eighteen to twenty-four year follow-up after complete rupture of the anterior cruciate ligament. Am J Sports Med 1996;27(6):711–7.

[12] Zeiss J, Paley K, Murray K, et al. Comparison of bone contusion seen by MRI in partial and complete tears of the anterior cruciate ligament. J Comput Assist Tomogr 1995;19:773–6.

[13] O'Neill DB. Arthroscopic assisted reconstruction of the anterior cruciate ligament. J Bone Joint Surg 2001;83A(9):1329–32.

[14] Shirakura K, Terauchi M, Kizuki S, Moro S, Kimura M. The natural history of untreated anterior cruciate ligament tears in recreational athletes. Clin Orthop 1995;317:227–36.

[15] Ciccotti MG, Lombardo SJ, Nonweiler B, Pink M. Nonoperative treatment of ruptures of the anterior cruciate ligament in middle-aged patients. Results after long-term follow-up. J Bone Joint Surg 1994;76(A):1315–21.

[16] Jarvela T, Kannus P, Jarvinen M. Anterior cruciate ligament reconstruction in patients with or without accompanying injuries: A re-examination of subjects 5 to 9 years after reconstruction. Arthroscopy 2001;17(8):818–25.

[17] Otto D, Pinczewski LA, Clingeleffer A, Ross O. Five year results of single incision arthroscopic anterior cruciate ligament reconstruction with patellar tendon autograft. Am J Sports Med 1998;26(2):181–8.

[18] Ahmed A, Burke D. In vitro measurement of static pressure distribution in the synovial joints- Part 1: tibial surface of the knee. J Biomech Eng 1983;105:216–25.

[19] MacDonald P, Miniaci A, Fowler P, et al. A biomechanical analysis of joint contact forces in the posterior cruciate deficient knee. Knee Surg Sports Traumatol Arthrosc 1996;3(4):252–5.

[20] Fowler PJ, Messieh S. Isolated posterior cruciate ligament injuries in athletes. Am J Sports Med 1987;15:553–7.

[21] Clancy W, Shelbourn K, Zoellner G, et al. Treatment of knee joint instability secondary to rupture of the posterior cruciate ligament. Report of a new procedure. J Bone Joint Surg 1983; 65(3):310–22.

[22] Dejour H, Walch G, Peyrote J, et al. The natural history of rupture of the posterior cruciate ligament. Rev Chir Orthop Reparatrice Appar Mot 1988;74(1):35–43.

[23] Torg J, Barton T, Pavlov H. Natural history of the posterior cruciate deficient knee. Clin Orthop 1989;246:208–16.

[24] Shelbourne D, Davis T, Patel D. The natural history of acute, isolated nonoperatively treated posterior cruciate ligament injuries. Am J Sports Med 1999;27:276–83.

[25] Delee J, Drez D, Miller M. Orthopeadic sorts medicine; principles and practice. 2nd edition. Philadelphia: WB Saunders; 2003. p. 2094.

[26] Fairbank TJ. Knee joint changes after meniscectomy. J Bone Joint Surg Br 1948;30:664–70.

[27] Kettelkamp DB, Jacobs AW. Tibiofemoral contact area: determination and implications. J Bone Joint Surg Am 1972;54:349–56.

[28] Scheller G, Sobau C, Bulow JU. Arthroscopic partial lateral meniscectomy in an otherwise normal knee: clinical, functional, and radiographic results of a long-term follow-up study. Arthroscopy 2001;17(9):946–52.

[29] Schimmer RC, Brulhart KB, Claudio D, Glinz W. Arthroscopic partial meniscectomy: a 12-year follow-up and two-step evaluation of the long term course. Arthroscopy 1998;14(2):136–42.

[30] Buckwalter JA, Mow VC, Ratcliffe A. Restoration of injured or degenerated articular cartilage. J Am Acad Orthop Surg 1994;2:192–201.

[31] Fowler PJ. Bone bruises associated with anterior cruciate ligament disruption. Arthroscopy 1994;10:453–60.

[32] Shelbourne KD, Jari S, Gray T. Outcome of untreated traumatic articular cartilage defects of the knee. J Bone Joint Surg 2003;85A(2):8–16.

[33] Johnson DL, Urban WP, Caborn DNM, Vanarthos WJ, Carlson CS. Articular cartilage changes seen with magnetic resonance image detected bone bruises associated with acute anterior cruciate ligament rupture. Am J Sports Med 1998;26(3):409–14.

[34] Faber KJ, Dill JR, Amendola A, Thain L, Spouge A, Fowler PJ. Occult osteochondral lesions after anterior cruciate ligament rupture: six year magnetic resonance imaging follow-up study. Am J Sports Med 1999;27(4):489–94.

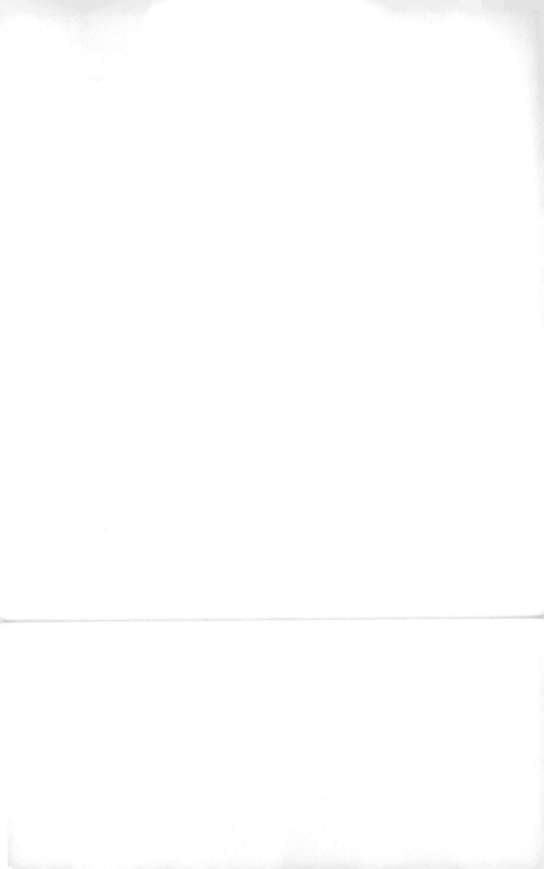

ELSEVIER
SAUNDERS

Clin Sports Med 24 (2005) 47–56

CLINICS
IN SPORTS
MEDICINE

Osteoarthritis Following Shoulder Instability

Robert H. Brophy, MD, MS[a,*], Robert G. Marx, MD[a,b]

[a]*Hospital for Special Surgery, 535 East 70th Street, New York, NY 10021, USA*
[b]*Weill Medical College of Cornell University, 525 East 68th Street, New York, NY 10021, USA*

Although dislocation of the shoulder is a common injury, estimated to occur in 0.5% to 1.7% [1,2] of individuals, the association between shoulder dislocation and the development of glenohumeral arthrosis has not been well studied or established in the literature. Rowe and others have discussed complications arising from shoulder dislocations; however, there was no mention of degenerative arthritis of the glenohumeral joint [3,4]. Considering the association between dislocation or recurrent instability and degenerative changes in other joints [5], it would appear reasonable to expect a similar relationship in the shoulder, especially considering the damage to cartilage and bone seen after traumatic shoulder dislocation [6].

Neer first recognized that a subset of patients with degenerative arthritis in the shoulder had a prior history of surgical repair for instability [7]. Samilson and Prieto [8] formally described the condition they called dislocation arthropathy of the shoulder, and noted such a finding even in patients with a single dislocation and no surgical intervention. Although there has been further research in this area, the understanding of this relationship is still evolving.

Incidence

The incidence of shoulder arthropathy in patients with shoulder instability is difficult to measure. Given that the majority of shoulder dislocations occur in

---

* Corresponding author.
E-mail address: brophyr@hss.edu (R.H. Brophy).

0278-5919/05/$ – see front matter © 2004 Elsevier Inc. All rights reserved.
doi:10.1016/j.csm.2004.08.010

younger patients [9], following such a population until the onset of degenerative arthritis is not feasible. Moreover, the long time period between dislocation and arthritis makes it difficult to control for other events in the interim. Adding to the complexity is the high rate of recurrence seen with shoulder dislocation, ranging from 10% to 90% after an initial dislocation [6,10–15].

There is no doubt that the humeral head suffers cartilage damage with shoulder dislocation. Taylor and Arciero [6] reported a series of 63 patients with first-time traumatic dislocations who were evaluated arthroscopically within 10 days of their dislocation. Osteochondral lesions of the humeral head were noted in 34 patients and chondral lesions were noted in an additional 23. Norlin [16] reported a series of 24 patients with first-time anterior shoulder dislocation assessed arthroscopically 1 to 3 days after injury. Osteochondral lesions were found in six shoulders, and the remaining 18 were all noted to have chondral lesions.

Cameron et al [17] reported on a series of 422 patients with a diagnosis of shoulder instability and no history of previous shoulder surgery who underwent an arthroscopic procedure. Chondral damage was rated according to the Outerbridge classification system. Of the 88 patients with acute instability (within 90 days of index injury to surgery, average 39.4 days after injury), 24% of the 88 had grade I or higher chondral lesions, 12% had Grade III or IV chondral damage. Of the 334 patients with chronic instability (more than 90 days from the initial injury to surgery and up to 29 years after injury, average 1129 days), 25% had grade I or higher chondral lesions and 12% had Grade III or IV lesions. Although there was no significant difference between patients with acute and chronic instability, there was a statistically significant association between the time from injury to surgery and the presence and grade of chondral damage with a linear trend between time from injury to surgery and the grade of chondral damage. The prevalence of grade III or IV lesions was reported as 15% in patients with anterior instability, 13% in patients with multidirectional instability, and 5% in patients with posterior instability, but the differences were not statistically significant. There was no control group in this study.

Hovelius et al [12] reported a prospective study of 247 first-time anterior shoulder dislocations in 245 patients aged 40 years or younger at the time of dislocation in which 11% of patients had radiographic evidence of mild arthrosis and 9% had radiographic evidence of moderate to severe arthrosis at 10-year follow-up evaluation (Fig. 1). Some patients with only a single dislocation were found to have arthrosis, and the incidence of arthrosis was found to be the same in patients with a single recurrence as in those with multiple dislocations or operative intervention for instability. The authors did not comment on whether patients showed clinical symptoms of shoulder osteoarthritis or if any patients underwent shoulder arthroplasty during the 10-year follow-up.

Neer et al [7] reported that 10% of their series of 273 total shoulder replacements for advanced osteoarthritis were in shoulders with a history of instability, although most of these had undergone previous surgery. Samilson and Prieto [8] described 74 shoulders in 70 patients with radiographic evidence of glenohumeral arthropathy and a history of single or multiple dislocations. They

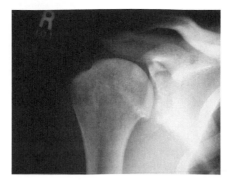

Fig. 1. Osteoarthritis in shoulder of patient with a history of shoulder dislocation.

did not find a significant correlation between the severity of arthrosis and the number of dislocations or a history of surgical treatment for instability, although the severity of arthrosis was associated with limitation of external rotation. A history of posterior dislocation was more common in the shoulders with more severe arthrosis. Gartsman et al [18] reported a series of 83 total shoulder replacements, with six patients (7.2%) reporting a history of instability.

Marx et al [19] investigated the relationship between shoulder dislocation and arthrosis with a case–control study. A total of 91 patients with glenohumeral arthritis who underwent hemi or total shoulder arthroplasty for osteoarthritis were compared with 282 patients without any history of shoulder symptoms who had undergone total knee arthroplasty. Patients with a history of previous shoulder dislocation were found to have a 19 times greater risk of developing severe shoulder arthrosis than patients who did not have such a history. When patients with a history of shoulder surgery before arthroplasty were excluded, patients had a 10-fold increased risk of developing arthrosis ($P = 0.003$). This analysis did not include the direction of the dislocation.

Matsoukis et al [20] reported on 55 shoulders that had a history of previous anterior dislocation out of a total of 1542 primary total shoulder replacements over 7 years. Of these 55 shoulders, 27 had previously undergone surgery to stabilize the joint while 28 had not undergone any shoulder surgery before the arthroplasty. The authors commented that they did not find any difference between shoulders previously treated with stabilizing surgery and those treated nonoperatively.

To summarize the available data, it is clear that some degree of chondral damage is associated with instability. The articular pathology is likely to worsen with time, although how quickly and in which patients is not well defined. There does appear to be an increased risk of developing symptomatic osteoarthritis and ultimately requiring a shoulder arthroplasty in patients with a history of instability, but again, more study is needed. The other important question is how, if at all, does surgical treatment for instability impact the risk for and progression of glenohumeral osteoarthritis in these patients?

Association of arthrosis with surgical treatment for instability

Surgical procedures to correct instability are known to put patients at risk for glenohumeral arthritis. The open Bankart, Bristow, Latarjet, Max Lange, Putti-Platt, and other procedures have all been shown to be associated with a risk for glenohumeral arthritis [8,21–28], particularly if the patient loses significant external rotation (Fig. 2).

Brems [9] identifies several factors that may contribute to the development of osteoarthritis after surgical treatment for instability. Inappropriate diagnosis of the direction and degree of instability can lead to a surgical procedure that may not be ideal for a given patient's (true) pathology. Not all instabilities are necessarily anterior or unidirectional. Even with the correct diagnosis, selection of a less optimal procedure perhaps due to surgeon preference, what Brems terms "The Standard Procedure for All," may factor in the subsequent development of arthrosis. Performing the procedure on the wrong side of the joint predisposes to excessive tightness and ultimately arthritis. Intraarticular metal hardware can contribute to the development of osteoarthritis [28]. Finally, the long-term implications of the increasingly popular arthroscopic stabilization instead of open procedures that have a longer track record is yet to be determined. Although the hope is for better long-term outcomes, there is always the risk of unforeseen complicating issues, including an unknown impact on the risk of developing osteoarthritis.

Patients have been known to develop osteoarthritis in both the early and late postoperative periods following surgical treatment for instability [29]. Early postoperative osteoarthritis is often related to hardware [28]. In the series presented by Zuckerman and Matsen, 21 out of 37 patients who developed arthritis of the shoulder were noted to have an instability repair using screws, and an additional 14 patients had undergone instability surgery using staples. Problems developed even in some patients with properly positioned hardware. Metal hardware may break or migrate [30], and thus contribute to osteoarthritic changes (Fig. 3). Early postoperative osteoarthritis ultimately resulting in total shoulder arthroplasty has also been seen after intraarticular extension of a pos-

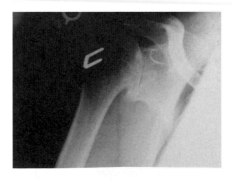

Fig. 2. Patient developed glenohumeral osteoarthritis after previous treatment for shoulder instability.

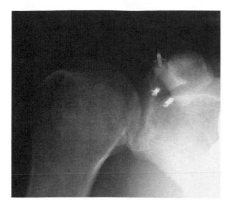

Fig. 3. Suture anchor loose within glenohumeral joint after treatment for shoulder instability.

terior glenoid osteotomy for recurrent posterior instability [31]. If a glenoid osteotomy is necessary, the cut should be made 6 [32] to 10 mm [33] from the articular margin. Bone block procedures have also been associated with the development of osteoarthritis [34,35], probably as a result of impingement on the articular cartilage.

Later onset of shoulder osteoarthritis after instability surgery is associated with excessive restriction of motion [29]. Hawkins and Angelo [21] described a series of 10 patients (11 shoulders) seen an average of 16.8 years after the Putti-Platt procedure with severe degenerative changes. They ascribed the development of osteoarthritis in these shoulders to an excessively tight repair, resulting in altered biomechanics of the glenohumeral joint, generating compression and shear forces on the articular surface. The series of Samilson and Prieto [8] included nine patients who underwent a Putti-Platt procedure, as well as six patients who developed osteoarthritis after a Magnuson-Stack repair, and two after a Bankart repair. They did not report the interval between instability surgery and the diagnosis of arthrosis, but they did note the time from initial dislocation to radiologic diagnosis of arthrosis ranged from 1 to 50 years.

The association between surgical treatment for instability and the subsequent development of osteoarthritis has been demonstrated. But again, rigorous data is lacking. Which patients are at risk and after which procedures? What is the impact of newer arthroscopic procedures on the risk of developing osteoarthritis? Perhaps most importantly, how does surgery change the pathogenesis of osteoarthritis compared with no surgical intervention? Also, the clinical significance of chondral changes following dislocation is unknown.

Significance of osteoarthritis after shoulder instability

The presence of glenohumeral osteoarthritis, particularly on radiograph, does not necessarily translate into clinically significant osteoarthritis. In the 10-year followup presented by Hovelius et al [12], the only comment on the clinical significance of arthropathy seen radiographically is that the "... patient's subjective assessment of function of the shoulder did not differ significantly..." between the shoulders with and without arthropathy. In the series presented by Cameron et al [17], the authors did not comment on the clinical significance, if any, of the osteoarthritis seen during arthroscopy. The case control study by Marx evaluated patients with arthritis severe enough to require total shoulder arthroplasty. Others have reported on patients who underwent total shoulder arthroplasty and who were noted to have a history of instability or dislocation. More long-term studies are clearly needed to define the relationship between the early onset of radiographically or arthroscopically diagnosed arthritic changes and clinically significant osteoarthritis.

Treatment of osteoarthritis after shoulder instability

Treatment for osteoarthrosis after shoulder instability depends on the presentation and etiology of the condition. If metal or a bone block impinging on the articular surface is noticed early, it may be possible to revise before the development of severe arthritis. Arthroscopic debridement, or an arthroscopic or open release in a patient with limited external rotation, are viable options if the patient presents early. Patients who present with advanced osteoarthritis are most often treated with total shoulder replacement if indicated, even in patients presenting at a relatively young age.

If the osteoarthritis is not too advanced, or if the symptoms are mostly mechanical, arthroscopic debridement may be performed [29]. If limited motion is the chief complaint, arthroscopic or open release can provide increased motion and a good result in patients with limited degenerative changes [29,36,37]. The series reported by McDonald et al [38] included 10 patients who developed mild to severe osteoarthritic changes in the glenohumeral joint following an anterior repair for recurrent dislocation. They were treated with release of the subscapularis and noted to have increased external rotation and relief of pain at an average follow-up of 3.5 years. Brems [9] described arthritis of dislocation as an entity presenting in young patients (average age 38) [39] with severe pain and restricted activity. He advocates shoulder arthroplasty (total or hemi based on the condition of the glenoid) as the appropriate treatment once the joint cartilage has been destroyed even in the face of young age. Most authors agree that advanced pain and degenerative change in patients with a history of instability or dislocation warrants shoulder arthroplasty, usually total.

Neer reported excellent or satisfactory results in 17 of 18 patients treated with total shoulder replacement for "arthritis of recurrent dislocation" evaluated at least 24 months after arthroplasty [7]. Young and Rockwood [36] noted relief of pain and functional ROM in all four patients who underwent total shoulder arthroplasty for osteoarthritis following a Bristow procedure for instability. Bigliani et al [40] reported 13 satisfactory results in a series of 17 patients who underwent shoulder replacement for osteoarthritis after surgery for instability. Sperling et al [41] reported on 31 shoulders in 31 patients with a mean age of 46 years who underwent arthroplasty, 21 total and 10 hemi, for osteoarthritis after instability surgery. Patients noted significant pain relief and improved external rotation and active abduction postoperatively. Eight of the total shoulder arthroplasty patients and three of the hemiarthroplasty patients required revision surgery.

Green and Norris [22] reviewed a series of patients with glenohumeral arthritis and found 39 patients with a history of instability or dislocation, of whom 19 had undergone surgical treatment for anterior instability. Of these 19 patients, 17 underwent shoulder arthroplasty (15 total and 2 hemi). Eleven patients required anterior soft tissue release at the time of arthroplasty (Fig. 4), and four had severe glenoid wear requiring surgical correction. Sixteen of the 17 shoulders were noted to improve after arthroplasty. Three shoulders were noted to require revision after the index arthroplasty.

Matsoukis et al [20] reported on the results of total shoulder arthroplasty in 55 shoulders with a prior anterior shoulder dislocation. Significant improvements in Constant score and ROM were reported, and 50 patients rated the result of their surgery as good or excellent. However, the outcomes were not as good as in patients with primary osteoarthritis. Patients who underwent total shoulder arthroplasty were noted to have a better outcome than patients who underwent hemiarthroplasty. No significant differences were found between shoulders with prior surgical treatment for instability and shoulders without prior surgical treatment.

In general, total shoulder replacement is an appropriate treatment for advanced osteoarthritis arising in shoulders with a history of instability. Outcomes are good, although not as good as in patients with primary osteoarthritis [20,22,40]. Contracture of the anterior soft tissue and erosion of the posterior glenoid are

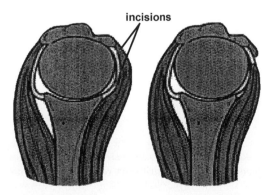

Fig. 4. Anterior soft tissue release during total shoulder arthroplasty (*From* Marx RG, Craig EV. Primary arthroplasty of the shoulder. In: Chapman MW, et al, editors. Chapman's orthopaedic surgery. 3rd edition. Philadelphia: Lippincott Williams & Wilkins; 2001. p. 2629–64; with permission.)

more common and more severe in patients with a history of previous instability surgery than patients with a history of primary osteoarthritis [9,22,40]. These patients also face a risk of higher rates of revision arthroplasty [41].

Summary

The relationship between shoulder instability and subsequent glenohumeral osteoarthritis has yet to be clearly defined. There does appear to be an increased risk of osteoarthritis in patients with shoulder instability that tends to occur at a younger age. However, the exact nature of that risk and the clinical implications remain unclear. There is no evidence to support shoulder stabilization surgery for the purpose of preventing glenohumeral osteoarthritis. Patients who develop symptomatic osteoarthritis with soft tissue contracture after instability surgery may benefit from debridement or soft tissue release early, although shoulder arthroplasty is the definitive treatment of choice for advanced symptomatic disease. Arthroplasty is generally successful, although the outcomes are not as satisfactory as in primary osteoarthritis.

References

[1] Hovelius L. Incidence of shoulder dislocation in Sweden. Clin Orthop 1982;166:127–31.
[2] Milgrom C, Mann G, Finestone A. A prevalence study of recurrent shoulder dislocations in young adults. J Shoulder Elbow Surg 1998;7:621–4.
[3] Rowe CR. Prognosis in dislocation of the shoulder. J Bone Joint Surg 1956;38A:957–77.
[4] Kazar B, Relovsky E. Prognosis of primary dislocation of the shoulder. Acta Orthop Scand 1969;40:216–24.
[5] Beaty JH. Orthopaedic knowledge update 6. Rosemont (IL): American Academy of Orthopaedic Surgeons; 1999.
[6] Taylor DC, Arciero RA. Pathologic changes associated with shoulder dislocations. Arthroscopic and physical examination findings in first-time, traumatic anterior dislocations. Am J Sports Med 1997;25:306–11.
[7] Neer CS, Watson KC, Stanton FJ. Recent experience in total shoulder replacement. J Bone Joint Surg 1982;64A:319–37.
[8] Samilson RL, Prieto V. Dislocation arthropathy of the shoulder. J Bone Joint Surg 1983; 65A:456–60.
[9] Brems JJ. Arthritis of dislocation. Orthop Clin North Am 1998;29:453–66.
[10] Hovelius L. Shoulder dislocation in Swedish ice hockey players. Am J Sports Med 1978;6: 373–7.
[11] Hovelius L. Anterior dislocation of the shoulder in teen-agers and young adults. Five-year prognosis. J Bone Joint Surg Am 1987;69:393–9.
[12] Hovelius L, Augustini BG, Fredin H, Johansson O, Norlin R, Thorling J. Primary anterior dislocation of the shoulder in young patients. A ten-year prospective study. J Bone Joint Surg Am 1996;78:1677–84.
[13] Hovelius L, Eriksson K, Fredin H, Hagberg G, Hussenius A, Lind B, et al. Recurrences after initial dislocation of the shoulder. Results of a prospective study of treatment. J Bone Joint Surg Am 1983;65:343–9.

[14] Kazar B, Relovszky E. Prognosis of primary dislocation of the shoulder. Acta Orthop Scand 1969;40:216–24.

[15] Simonet WT, Melton III LJ, Cofield RH, Ilstrup DM. Incidence of anterior shoulder dislocation in Olmsted County, Minnesota. Clin Orthop 1984;186:186–91.

[16] Norlin R. Intraarticular pathology in acute, first-time anterior shoulder dislocation: an arthroscopic study. Arthroscopy 1993;9:546–9.

[17] Cameron ML, Kocher MS, Briggs KK, Horan MP, Hawkins RJ. The prevalence of glenohumeral osteoarthrosis in unstable shoulders. Am J Sports Med 2003;31:53–5.

[18] Gartsman GM, Roddey TS, Hammerman SM. Shoulder arthroplasty with or without resurfacing of the glenoid in patients who have osteoarthritis. J Bone Joint Surg Am 2000;72:1193–7.

[19] Marx RG, McCarty EC, Montemurno TD, Altcheck DW, Craig EV, Warren RF. Development of arthrosis following dislocation of the shoulder: a case–control study. J Shoulder Elbow Surg 2002;11:1–5.

[20] Matsoukis J, Tabib W, Guiffault P, Mandelbaum A, Walch G, Nemoz C, et al. Shoulder arthroplasty in patients with a prior anterior shoulder dislocation: results of a multicenter study. J Bone Joint Surg 2003;85A:1417–24.

[21] Hawkins RJ, Angelo RL. Glenohumeral osteoarthritis: a late complication of the Putti-Platt repair. J Bone Joint Surg 1990;72A:1193–7.

[22] Green A, Norris TR. Shoulder arthroplasty for advanced glenohumeral arthritis after anterior instability repair. J Shoulder Elbow Surg 2001;10(6):539–45.

[23] Morrey BF, Janes JM. Recurrent anterior dislocation of the shoulder: long-term follow-up of the Putti-Platt and Bankart procedures. J Bone Joint Surg 1976;58A:252–6.

[24] O'Driscoll SW, Evans DC. Long-term results after staple capsulorrhaphy for anterior instability of the shoulder. J Bone Joint Surg 1993;75A:249–58.

[25] Rosenberg BN, Richmond JC, Levine WN. Long-term follow-up of Bankart reconstruction: incidence of late degenerative glenohumeral arthrosis. Am J Sports Med 1995;23:538–44.

[26] Singer GC, Kirkland PM, Emery RJ. Coracoid transposition for recurrent anterior instability of the shoulder. A 20-year follow up study. J Bone Joint Surg Br 1995;77B:73–6.

[27] Trevelyn DW, Richardson MW, Fanelli GC. Degenerative joint disease following extracapsular anterior shoulder reconstruction. Contemp Orthop 1992;25:151–6.

[28] Zuckerman JD, Matsen III FA. Complications about the glenohumeral joint related to the use of screws and staples. J Bone Joint Surg 1984;66A:175–80.

[29] Wall MS, Warren RF. Complications of shoulder instability surgery. Clin Sports Med 1995; 14:973–1000.

[30] Lyons FA, Rockwood CA. Migration of pins used in operations on the shoulder. J Bone Joint Surg 1990;72A:1262–7.

[31] Johnston GH, Hawkins RJ, Haddad R, et al. A complication of posterior glenoid osteotomy for recurrent posterior shoulder instability. Clin Orthop 1984;187:147–9.

[32] Scott Jr DJ. Treatment of recurrent posterior dislocation of the shoulder by glenoplasty. Report of three cases. J Bone Joint Surg Am 1967;49A:471–6.

[33] English E, Macnab I. Recurrent posterior dislocation of the shoulder. Can J Surg 1974;17: 147–51.

[34] Hindmarsh J, Lindberg A. Eden-Hybbinette's operation for recurrent dislocation of the humeroscapular joint. Acta Orthop Scand 1967;38:459–78.

[35] Rockwood Jr CA, Gerber C. Analysis of failed surgical procedures for anterior shoulder instability. Orthop Trans 1985;9:48.

[36] Young CD, Rockwood CA. Complications of a failed Bristow procedure and their management. J Bone Joint Surg 1991;73A:969–81.

[37] Steinman SR, Flatow EL, Pollock RG, Glasgow MD, Bigliani LU. Evaluation and surgical treatment of failed shoulder instability repairs. Orthop Trans 1992;16:727.

[38] MacDonald PB, Hawkins RJ, Fowler PJ, Miniaci A. Release of the subscapularis for internal rotation contracture and pain after anterior repair for recurrent anterior dislocation of the shoulder. J Bone Joint Surg Am 1992;74:734–7.

[39] Brems JJ. Shoulder replacement in arthritis of dislocation. Orthoped Trans 1989;13:235.

[40] Bigliani LU, Weinstein DM, Glasgow MT, Pollock RG, Flatow EL. Glenohumeral arthroplasty for arthritis after instability surgery. J Shoulder Elbow Surg 1995;4(2):87–94.

[41] Sperling JW, Antuna SA, Sanchez-Sotelo J, Schleck C, Cofield RH. Shoulder arthroplasty for arthritis after instability surgery. J Bone Joint Surg 2002;84A(10):1775–81.

ELSEVIER
SAUNDERS

Clin Sports Med 24 (2005) 57–70

CLINICS
IN SPORTS
MEDICINE

Osteoarthritis in Other Joints (Hip, Elbow, Foot, Ankle, Toes, Wrist) after Sports Injuries

Jason Koh, MD[a],*, Jeffrey Dietz, MD[b]

[a]Department of Orthopaedic Surgery, Northwestern University Medical Center, 675 N. St. Clair, Galter 17-100, Chicago, IL 60611, USA
[b]Northwestern Feinberg School of Medicine, Orthopaedic Surgery, 645 N. Michigan Ave., Suite 910, Chicago, IL 60611, USA

Osteoarthritis of nonknee joints, although less common than knee osteoarthritis, remains a significant and disabling condition for many present and former athletes. These injuries can be caused by repeated loads or following a specific traumatic event. The resulting pain and loss of motion can limit function and ability. Arthroscopic techniques in many cases enables surgeons to symptomatically treat limitations of range of motion and pain, prolonging active careers. Joint replacement remains the ultimate solution for hip osteoarthritis, and may be a viable option in ankle osteoarthritis.

Osteoarthritis of the hip is relatively common in athletes, second only to osteoarthritis of the knee. It may be the result of chronic overuse or secondary to specific traumatic events, such as transient subluxation or chondral injury [1]. At present, treatment options are limited, but the expanding use of arthroscopic techniques may provide a minimally invasive means of treating impinging osteophytes or performing articular cartilage transplantation.

Etiology

Osteoarthritis of the hip in athletes is typically the result of cumulative overuse, without specific injury in the majority of cases. Specific risk factors include high loads, sudden or irregular impact [2], and preexisting abnormalities such as

* Corresponding author.
 E-mail address: Kohj1@hotmail.com (J. Koh).

0278-5919/05/$ – see front matter © 2004 Elsevier Inc. All rights reserved.
doi:10.1016/j.csm.2004.08.011
sportsmed.theclinics.com

dysplasia [3,4]. Recently, labral tears of the hip have been implicated in early osteoarthritis [5]. Multiple studies have demonstrated a risk of hip osteoarthritis for professional soccer players that may be as high as 13.2%, or 10.2 times that of the general population, even in the absence of identifiable injury to the joint [6–8]. Other studies have shown other significant increases in risk in rugby players [9,10], javelin throwers [11], high jumpers, track, and field sports [12]. Hip arthritis is common among former National Football League (NFL) players, with 55.6% reporting some arthritic problem in a 2001 NFL Player's Association Survey [13,14]. The association of hip osteoarthritis with significant athletic activity has been demonstrated in female as well as male athletes [15–18].

It is unclear whether running is a risk factor for hip osteoarthritis. The literature is significantly divided, with data demonstrating that running or track and field events increase risk [19,20], make no difference [21–23], or are even potentially protective [24,25]. Biomechanical abnormalities or trauma may contribute to abnormal loading forces at the joint, but uninjured, nondysplastic runners may not be at increased risk. At this point, no definitive conclusions can be made with regard to this activity.

Another cause of hip osteoarthritis is as the sequelae of avascular necrosis of the hip. This can be traumatic, idiopathic, or possibly related to steroid use. Avascular necrosis can be the result of transient hip subluxation or dislocation disrupting the blood supply to the femoral head. A hematoma of the hip joint should be promptly decompressed to decrease the risk of avascular necrosis, which may occur from an increase in intracapsular pressure preventing blood flow to the femoral head [26]. Nontraumatic idiopathic avascular necrosis has also developed in athletes, resulting in early joint replacement. The use of corticosteroid medications may contribute to avascular necrosis in this patient population.

Symptoms

Primary complaints of hip osteoarthritis include pain and lack of range of motion. The athlete may not specifically complain of "pain" per se, but rather discomfort or stiffness. Often this is manifested as discomfort at start-up after being sedentary. Typically the patient has groin pain, which helps differentiate this from other causes of lower extremity pain including lumbar radiculopathy or greater trochanteric bursitis. On physical examination, loss of range of motion is common, particularly in internal rotation. Flexion is relatively well preserved until late in the disease. Standard radiographic findings include loss of joint space, marginal osteophytes, sclerosis, cysts, or in late stages incongruity of the joint.

Treatment

Typical nonsurgical management includes the use of analgesic or anti-inflammatory medication, alteration of level of activity, and gentle physical therapy designed to improve range of motion. Other interventions such as intraarticular injection of corticosteroid may provide temporary pain relief [27] similar to that found in the knee. Anecdotal reports have been presented on the use of hyaluronic acid injections in the hip; however, no peer-reviewed data is currently available. This is the subject of an ongoing multicenter clinical study.

Total joint replacement provides excellent function and pain relief. However, concerns remain about infection, dislocation, and wear. It is clear that wear is related to activity [28,29]. There have been several well-publicized cases of athletes who continued to participate in sports activity with subsequent need for early revision following joint replacement. Advances in bearing surface materials such as ceramics, metals, and polyethylene hold great promise for decreasing the rate of wear and hopefully the rate of revision.

Osteotomy has become an increasingly popular option in Europe for early arthritis [30]. Although not specifically described in athletes, pelvic and femoral osteotomies are performed in young adults to correct for femoroacetabular impingement and relieve hip pain [31,32]. These techniques may limit the progression of hip osteoarthritis, but are extremely technically difficult and carry a substantial risk of intraarticular fracture or other complications.

Hip arthroscopy is a minimally invasive procedure that can provide improvements in pain and function in athletes with arthritis. Using slightly modified arthroscopic equipment, unstable articular cartilage flaps, labral tears, loose bodies, and synovitis can be debrided from the joint. Focal articular cartilage defects can be treated with a microfracture procedure to stimulate formation of healing fibrocartilage.

A novel treatment for hip arthritis is the removal of impinging marginal osteophytes from the femoral head and neck to improve range of motion and decrease pain. Under a combination of arthroscopic and fluoroscopic guidance, the femoral head and neck can be reshaped to recreate the normal head–neck contour and avoid excessive femoroacetabular impingement, similar to the open technique developed by Ganz (Fig. 1). Associated labral tears and focal chondral defects are also be treated arthroscopically.

We typically perform hip arthroscopy in the supine position. Gentle traction is applied to the operative leg, and under fluoroscopic guidance a spinal needle is introduced into the joint from an anterior superior peritrochanteric portal. This is followed by placement of a flexible guidewire through the needle and then cannulated trocar and cannula over the wire. A second, anterior portal is created under a combination of fluoroscopic and arthroscopic visualization. Intraarticular pathology is debrided, including chondral flaps, labral tears, and microfracture for any exposed bone. The scope is then gently withdrawn to visualize the acetabular margin and the femoral head. A full radius shaver is used to debride prominent impinging osteophytic bone from the margins of the femoral head and neck under a combination of arthroscopic and fluoroscopic guidance.

Our short-term results for arthroscopic debridement and osteophyte resection have been promising (Fig. 2). Sixteen patients had an average improvement in range of motion of 10 degrees of abduction, 10 degrees of internal rotation,

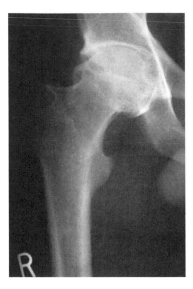

Fig. 1. Radiograph of 43-year-old active male with hip osteoarthritis. Note superior-lateral osteophyte that impinges in abduction.

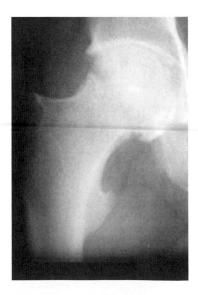

Fig. 2. Radiograph of patient after arthroscopic resection of superior-lateral osteophyte. Patient had improved abduction of 30 degrees.

5 degrees of flexion, and 5 degrees of external rotation. Visual analog scale pain scores decreased from 8 to 3. These patients have been able to return to high-level physical activity including firefighting, horseback riding, and soccer. Arthroscopic techniques may also eventually be a means of delivering scaffold-based articular cartilage repair.

Osteoarthritis of the elbow and wrist

Osteoarthritis of the elbow

Osteoarthritis of the elbow may be secondary to repetitive overuse when skeletally mature as well as following trauma or after repetitive overload in adolescence, when osteochondritis dessicans of the capitellum may develop. The elbow undergoes tremendous stresses during such athletic activities as throwing [33]. Secondary changes such as the formation of posterior olecranon osteophytes, osteophyte formation in the olecranon fossa, coronoid osteophytes, loose bodies, and chondromalacia of the radius and capitellum are common, and may occur at a relatively young age, particularly in throwing athletes [34]. Long-term, osteoarthritic changes are seen in many throwing athletes [35].

Symptoms

Many athletes with radiographic and clinical evidence of osteoarthritis can continue to perform at a high level of professional activity. For example, asymptomatic loss of range of motion of the dominant arm is extremely common in professional pitchers. Symptomatic individuals may have loss of range of motion, pain at end range extension, intermittent locking secondary to loose bodies, or more general pain and swelling. Occasionally, ulnar nerve symptoms may be elicited secondary to osteophyte formation or instability. It is important to note that concomitant medial instability is seen in about 25% of throwing athletes with posterior elbow impingement [36]. In these cases, the posteromedial olecranon osteophyte forms in response to valgus extension overload stresses, and resection of the osteophyte may reveal underlying valgus instability. The standard clinical evaluation of these patients should include range of motion (flexion-extension and pronation-supination), the posterior impingement or "clunk" test performed by brisk extension eliciting pain, careful neurovascular examination, particularly in regard to the ulnar nerve, and evaluation for medial instability. Radiographic evaluation with a plain radiograph can include a "thrower's view" of the olecranon [37], which can help more clearly define a posteromedial osteophyte. This is performed with the elbow flexed 120 to 130 degrees and externally rotated 30 to 40 degrees on the plate. CT scans and magnetic resonance imaging can also demonstrate olecranon and coronoid osteophytes.

Treatment

Initial management consists of nonsteroidal anti-inflammatory drugs and heat or ice applied to the elbow. A light compressive dressing or brace often will provide some subjective support to the elbow and keep the joint warm. Gentle stretching and warm up before activity is also helpful.

If further treatment is indicated, debridement has proven to be extremely effective in returning athletes to a high level of function [36,38,39]. Although technically challenging, one can arthroscopically remove loose bodies in the elbow, perform chondroplasty and osteophyte resection, capsular release, and even radial head resection [40–42]. We perform elbow arthroscopy with the patient in the lateral position with the arm over a post. This allows easy access to the posterior compartment where the majority of the procedure is typically conducted. A tourniquet is applied and the capsule distended by injection of fluid into the posterolateral soft spot formed by the triangle of the radial head, lateral epicondyle, and olecranon tip. Neurovascular structures are identified and the anterior compartment is entered from either the anteromedial or anterolateral portal. Evaluation of the anterior compartment is completed, along with resection of impinging coronoid osteophytes and removal of loose bodies. Occasionally, if there are significant capsular contractures, the anterior capsule is released from the humerus or divided proximally.

The posterior compartment is then entered via central trans-tricep portal and a portal along the lateral border of the triceps. The olecranon fossa is identified and defined, and cleared of loose bodies and osteophytes. The posterior tip of the olecranon is resected using a combination of motorized arthroscopic instruments and small osteotomes. In throwing athletes, great care is taken to resect only osteophytic tissue because excessive resection may result in destabilization of the elbow to valgus stress. If there is significant excessive osteophyte formation, an arthroscopic Outerbridge-Kashiwagi procedure can be performed.

Our experience with athletes who had painful impinging osteophytes has been very successful [36].

Forty-nine consecutive patients underwent arthroscopic debridement of posterior elbow over a period of 7 years. All patients experienced limitation of activity (severe, affecting activities of daily living, 6; partial activity only, 11 preventing sports, 32). Elbow pain was severe in 8, moderate 20, occasional 21. An elbow score was calculated, with mean score of 171 of 200, subjective component (pain, swelling, locking, activity) 73 of 100; objective (contracture, pronation/supination, sagittal arc) 88 of 100. At a mean of 43 (14–81) months follow-up pain improved in 47 patients (27 no pain, 20 occasional pain). Twenty-nine patients who had limited motion improved an average of 12°. Forty-five patients were able to return to their desired level of activity; 14 returned to professional sports, 7 to college, and 24 to high school or recreational sports activities. Average elbow score improved 20 points to 191 of 200; subjective 94, objective 97.

Osteoarthritis of the wrist

Primary osteoarthritis of the wrist is rare. Most cases of radiocarpal arthritis are secondary to structural changes that are often precipitated by trauma. Traumatic injuries to the wrist are a common entity in the athletic population. In a study by Rettig et al from the The Methodist Sports Clinic, approximately 3% of all sports injuries seen involved the wrist or hand [43]. The natural history of many of these injuries involves the development of arthritis at the radiocarpal, distal radioulnar joint, or intercarpal joint surfaces. This review will focus on degenerative pathology of the wrist in the athletic population after such trauma.

Scapholunate advanced collapse

Scapholunate interosseous ligament injury is the most common form of carpal instability [44]. It results from excessive wrist extension and ulnar deviation common in collision and contact sports [45]. Clinical diagnosis is suggested by symptoms such as dorsoradial wrist pain and weakness in grasp. On examination patients have a hypermobile scaphoid that translates into a positive Watson or scaphoid shift sign.

Alterations of carpal kinetmatics that occur when the scapholunate ligament is disrupted can lead to the development of radiocarpal arthritis. Without a competent scapholunate ligament the scaphoid falls into a flexed position, while the lunate and triquetrum extend. This position is referred to as dorsal intercalated segmental instability [46,47]. This pattern of instability significantly alters the articular contact areas and stress patterns within the carpus, particularly the scaphoid. Biomechanical studies by Burgess et al showed a 45% reduction in radioscaphoid contact area with 5 degrees of scaphoid flexion [48]. Scapholunate advanced collapse progresses in a staged fashion. Stage 1 consists of degeneration of the radial styloid and proximal pole of the scaphoid. Stage 2 involves the proximal pole of the scaphoid and scaphoid fossa. In stage 3, the capitate migrates between the scaphoid and the lunate resulting in capitolunate degeneration, and stage 4 includes pancarpal arthritis.

Once degenerative changes are seen within the radiocarpal joint salvage-type procedures become the mainstay of treatment. Procedures most commonly performed are scaphoid excision with four corner fusion and proximal row carpectomy. With both the four corner fusion and the proximal row carpectomy, there is a loss of approximately 50% of wrist motion in the flexion/extension plane and 20% loss of grip strength. The deficit leaves the athlete with approximately 30 to 40 degrees of both wrist flexion and extension, but does not appear to limit most sports related activities [49]. However, proximal row carpectomy is limited to patients who have no evidence of degenerative changes seen within the midcarpal joint. The later stages of advanced collapse may require more extensive fusion procedures such as wirst arthrodesis, which would severely limit motion and ability to compete.

Scaphoid nonunion advanced collapse

Scaphoid fractures account for almost 70% of all fractures of the carpal bones, and are the most common carpal fracture within the population between 15 and 30 [50]. The fracture results from a fall on the hand with the wrist dorsiflexed greater than 90 degrees, and can occur during active participation in sports. Reister et al estimated that approximately 1 out of every 100 college football players will sustain a fracture of the scaphoid [51].

Anatomic considerations are of paramount importance during evaluation of scaphoid fractures. The vascular supply to the scaphoid is predominantly from a branch of the radial artery, which enters the nonarticular portion of the scaphoid on its dorsal ridge [52]. The proximal pole of the scaphoid receives its bloody supply through retrograde flow, and fractures that occur proximal to the insertion of the vascular supply have a high rate of nonunion.

The natural history of scaphoid nonunion is the development of radiocarpal arthritis in the majority of patients [53,54]. This phenomenon is related to the biomechanics of the carpal bones of the proximal row. An unstable scaphoid fracture is subject to the forces exerted upon its fragments by the intercarpal and radiocarpal ligaments. A resultant apex dorsal angulation through the fracture, or a so-called humback deformity, occurs with time. This deformity causes an alteration in kinetmatics of the proximal row similar to that seen in scapholunate advance collapse. The carpus falls into a dorsal intercalated segmental instability pattern, and progressive radiocarpal arthrosis ensues. Treatment options for scaphoid nonunion advanced collapse are identical to those performed in scapholunate advanced collapse. The only notable difference is the need to address the fracture nonunion usually with bone graft and some variety of internal fixation.

Radiocarpal arthritis after intraarticular distal radius fractures

Distal radius fractures are common in young athletes, and can occur during any sport where the athlete falls on an outstretched hand. Unlike fractures in the older population, fractures in young patients tend to be higher energy injuries, and more frequently are intrarticular. Further, it has been shown that nearly all intrarticular fractures that are displaced over 2 mm go on to develop posttraumatic arthritis if the articular surface is not adequately restored [55]. Knirk et al evaluated displaced intraarticular distal radius fractures in young active patients and found that 65% of the patients had developed radiographic evidence of radiocarpal arthritis at a mean follow up of 7.1 years despite method of treatment. The factor that most strongly correlated to degeneration of the joint was residual displacement at time of union [56]. Catalano et al also showed a high rate of osteoarthritis in a similar population, but found that function impairment was not as significant as was predicted based on radiographic evaluation [57]. Therefore, it is recommended that salvage type procedures be reserved for patients with severe pain and loss of function rather than mere radiographic evidence of osteoarthritis.

Distal radioulnar joint arthritis

A common source of ulnar sided wrist pain in athletes is pathology at the distal radioulnar joint. Traumatic events usually involve axial loading and rotational stress from a fall onto an outstretched hand. This mechanism of injury is common in hockey, raquet players, water skiing, and pole vaulting [58]. Traumatic injuries to the distal radioulnar joint can lead to chronic instability, alterations of contact stresses, and subsequent arthritis. Instability can be determined clinically the piano key sign.

When the athlete begins to develop degenerative changes within the distal radioulnar joint they may complain of persistent activity related ulnar sided wrist pain. On examination, if the ulnar and radius are compressed at the wrist and the forearm is rotated, a grind test is elicited [59]. Conservative therapy is always attempted in these athletes, but continued pain may require resectional arthroplasty. Historically, the Darrach excisional arthroplasty has been the workhorse for surgical management of distal radioulnar joint arthritis; however, following this procedure, high-demand athletes may experience persistent instability of the distal ulna as well as mechanical symptoms such as clicking or snapping. For this reason, some authors prefer to maintain the integrity of the triangular fibrocartilage complex and, thus, the stability of the ulnar side of the wrist using a matched hemiresection arthroplasty described by Watson [60].

Pisotriquetral arthritis

Racquet sports aggravate pisotriquetral inflammation secondary to repetitive wrist flexion and direct compression on the joint. Differentiating the etiology of ulnar side wrist pain can be difficult. Therefore, clinical examination will confirm diagnosis including pain with direct manipulation of the pisiform is common. If diagnosis is still in question lidocaine can be injected at the pisotriquetral articulation. Diagnosis can be confirmed radiographically with the wrist in 30 degrees of supination, which provides the best view of the articular surface of the pisiform. Conservative management is recommended in early stages consisting of immobilization and nonsteroidal antiinflammatory medications. If the patient fails conservative management, surgical excision of the pisiform can be performed reliably with limited functional impairment [61,62].

Osteoarthritis of the ankle and foot

Osteoarthritis of the ankle

Osteoarthritis of the ankle is characterized by the formation of impinging bone spurs, loose bodies, and joint space narrowing. Anterior ankle impingement secondary to anterior osteophytes ("footballer's ankle" [63]) may be caused secondary to repeated high dorsiflexion loads at the ankle. Other proposed etiologies include anterior capsular strain and traction [64]. These lesions can restrict range of motion, particularly dorsiflexion, and may also cause pain. Osteoarthritis of the ankle is more common in professional soccer players [7] and ballet dancers [64] but not significantly so in high jumpers [65]. We have also observed similar, often asymptomatic, radiographic findings in professional football and baseball players.

Scranton and McDermott [66] have developed a classification scheme for anterior osteophyte formation: Stage I—anterior tibial osteophytes less than 3 mm, Stage II—osteophytes greater than 3 mm with osteochondral reaction, Stage III—tibial and talar kissing lesions, Stage IV—global arthritis.

Ankle arthroscopy for anterior ankle debridement has proven to be very successful in many cases, particularly in the athletic population. Several authors have reported excellent results, and Pierce and Scranton have reported that the arthroscopic debridement had shorter length of hospitalization and time to recovery. Grade IV patients were not suitable for arthroscopic debridement. Return to sports occurs in an average of 4 months in 10 of 13 athletes in one study [67]. van Dijk and coauthors indicated that the degree of osteoarthritic changes is a better prognostic factor for the outcome of arthroscopic surgery for anterior ankle impingement than size and location of the spurs [68].

In arthroscopic ankle debridement standard anterior portals are created. Conducting the procedure without traction may improve visualization because traction may pull the anterior capsule against the osteophytes anteriorly. Debridement is performed using arthroscopic shavers or burrs [69].

Ankle fusion is considered to be the standard solution for severe ankle arthritis. We recommend a trial with a boot or cast limiting ankle motion to evaluate how well it is tolerated. The results of ankle fusion long term are significant, however, and many patients will develop pain and functional limitations from ipsilateral foot arthritis [70]. Ankle replacement may prevent some of these problems [71].

Treatment

Treatment of ankle arthritis initially should consist of analgesic medication, nonsteroidal antiinflammatory medcations, physical therapy, and local modalities. Many patients will respond well to this treatment, however.

Osteoarthritis of the great toe

Hallux rigidus

Hallux rigidus is most common deformity of the first metatarsal phalangeal joint in the athlete. It lies at the end of the spectrum of hyperextension injuries to the metatarsal phalangeal (MTP) of the great toe. With this mechanism, the foot is typically in a dorsiflexed position with the forefoot on the ground and the heel raised. An external force drives the first MTP joint into an exaggerated position. Initially capsuloligamentous structures are stretched or rupture, and a "turf toe" injury occurs. With more extremes of hyperdorsiflexion, compression can occur across the articular cartilage leading to subchondral bone collapse and eventual degenerative changes of the joint [72]. Hyperextension injury to the first MTP joint is one of the most common mechanisms that can cause hallux rigidus. Bowers and Martin correlated the incidence of traumatic injuries to the MTP of the great toe with artificial surfaces and the use of more flexible shoewear [73]. This injury is common in football, but can occur in any athlete. Dancers may develop hallux rigidus secondary to trauma to the joint from positions requiring repetitive hyperdorsiflexion of the joint.

Diagnosis of hallux rigidus is usually obvious on physical examination. Patients complain of pain at the first MTP joint, dorsal prominence, and restricted dorsiflexion often less than 30 degrees. These symptoms can cause significant disability for the athlete. Normal walking requires approximately 65 to 75 degrees of dorsiflexion during the toe-off phase of gait and can be significantly increased for activities such as running and forward drive [74].

Treatment begins with conservative measures such as alterations in shoe wear and nonsteroidal medications. However, the natural history of the disease cannot be altered by these measures, and patients often require surgical management. Many surgical treatment options have been proposed, including cheilectomy, dorsiflexion osteotomy of the proximal phalanx, resection arthroplasty, implant arthroplasty, and arthrodesis. There is little literature available that directly compares these methods in an athletic population, but Mulier et al reported good or excellent results in 20 of 21 feet treated with cheilectomy. Furthermore, they contend that cheilectomy preserves a variable amount of motion or power that is lost with resection arthroplasty and arthrodesis, and it avoids the potential complications associated with these methods of treatment. However, they conceded that cheilectomy is not a suitable treatment for patients with advanced degenerative changes, and can be joint destructive [75]. Treatment, therefore, must be individualized to the patients disease as well as their needs and expectations.

References

[1] Olsen O, Vingard E, Koster M, Alfredsson L. Etiologic fractions for physical work load, sports and overweight in the occurrence of coxarthrosis. Scand J Work Environ Health 1994; 20(3):184–8.
[2] Kujala UM, Kaprio J, Sarna S. Osteoarthritis of weight bearing joints of lower limbs in former elite male athletes. BMJ 1994;308(6923):231–4.
[3] Leunig M, Casillas MM, Hamlet M, Hersche O, Notzli H, Slongo T, et al. Slipped capital femoral epiphysis: early mechanical damage to the acetabular cartilage by a prominent femoral metaphysis. Acta Orthop Scand 2000;71(4):370–5.
[4] Lequesne MG, Dang N, Lane NE. Sport practice and osteoarthritis of the limbs. Osteoarthritis Cartilage 1997;5(2):75–86.
[5] McCarthy JC, Noble PC, Schuck MR, Wright J, Lee J. The Otto E. Aufranc award: the role of labral lesions to development of early degenerative hip disease. Clin Orthop 2001;393:25–37.

[6] Shepard GJ, Banks AJ, Ryan WG. Ex-professional association footballers have an increased prevalence of osteoarthritis of the hip compared with age matched controls despite not having sustained notable hip injuries. Br J Sports Med 2003;37(1):80–1.

[7] Drawer S, Fuller C. Propensity for osteoarthritis and lower limb joint pain in retired professional soccer players. Br J Sports Med 2001;35:402–8.

[8] Lindberg H, Roos H, Gardsell P. Prevalence of coxarthrosis in former soccer players. 286 players compared with matched controls. Acta Orthop Scand 1993;64(2):165–7.

[9] Meir RA, McDonald KN, Russell R. Injury consequences from participation in professional rugby league: a preliminary investigation. Br J Sports Med 1997;31:132–4.

[10] Lequesne MG, Dang N, Lane NE. Sport practice and osteoarthritis of the limbs. Osteoarthritis Cartilage 1997;5(2):75–86.

[11] Schmitt H, Brocai DR, Lukoschek M. High prevalence of hip arthrosis in former elite javelin throwers and high jumpers: 41 athletes examined more than 10 years after retirement from competitive sports. Acta Orthop Scand 2004;75(1):34–9.

[12] Vingard E, Sandmark H, Alfredsson L. Musculoskeletal disorders in former athletes. A cohort study in 114 track and field champions. Acta Orthop Scand 1995;66(3):289–91.

[13] Callahan L. Osteoarthritis in retired National Football League (NFL) Players: The role of injuries and playing position. Abstract presentation: American College of Rheumatology Annual Meeting New Orleans (LA) October; 2002.

[14] http://www.medicalpost.com/mpcontent/article.jsp?content=/content/extract/rawart/3811/19a.html.

[15] Vingard E, Alfredsson L, Malchau H. Osteoarthrosis of the hip in women and its relation to physical load at work and in the home. Ann Rheum Dis 1997;56(5):293–8.

[16] Spector TD, Harris PA, Hart DJ, Cicuttini FM, Nandra D, Etherington J, et al. Risk of osteoarthritis associated with long-term weight-bearing sports: a radiologic survey of the hips and knees in female ex-athletes and population controls. Arthritis Rheum 1996;39(6):988–95.

[17] Vingard E, Alfredsson L, Malchau H. Osteoarthrosis of the hip in women and its relationship to physical load from sports activities. Am J Sports Med 1998;26(1):78–82.

[18] Lane NE, Hochberg MC, Pressman A, Scott JC, Nevitt MC. Recreational physical activity and the risk of osteoarthritis of the hip in elderly women. J Rheumatol 1999;26(4):849–54.

[19] Marti B, Knobloch M, Tschopp A, Jucker A, Howald H. Is excessive running predictive of degenerative hip disease? Controlled study of former elite athletes. BMJ 1989;299(6691):91–3.

[20] Vingard E, Alfredsson L, Goldie I, Hogstedt C. Sports and osteoarthrosis of the hip. An epidemiologic study. Am J Sports Med 1993;21(2):195–200.

[21] Panush RS, Schmidt C, Caldwell JR, Edwards NL, Longley S, Yonker R, et al. Is running associated with degenerative joint disease? JAMA 1986;255(9):1152–4.

[22] Konradsen L, Hansen EM, Sondergaard L. Long distance running and osteoarthrosis. Am J Sports Med 1990;18(4):379–81.

[23] Lane NE, Oehlert JW, Bloch DA, Fries JF. The relationship of running to osteoarthritis of the knee and hip and bone mineral density of the lumbar spine: a 9 year longitudinal study. J Rheumatol 1998;25(2):334–41.

[24] Kettunen JA, Kujala UM, Kaprio J, Koskenvuo M, Sarna S. Lower-limb function among former elite male athletes. Am J Sports Med 2001;29(1):2–8.

[25] Sohn RS, Micheli LJ. The effect of running on the pathogenesis of osteoarthritis of the hips and knees. Clin Orthop 1985;198:106–9.

[26] Moorman III CT, Warren RF, Hershman EB, Crowe JF, Potter HG, Barnes R, et al. Traumatic posterior hip subluxation in American football. J Bone Joint Surg Am 2003;85-A(7):1190–6.

[27] Plant MJ, Borg AA, Dziedzic K, Saklatvala J, Dawes PT. Radiographic patterns and response to corticosteroid hip injection. Ann Rheum Dis 1997;56(8):476–80.

[28] Feller JA, Kay PR, Hodgkinson JP, Wroblewski BM. Activity and socket wear in the Charnley low-friction arthroplasty. J Arthroplasty 1994;9(4):341–5.

[29] Kilgus DJ, Dorey FJ, Finerman GA, Amstutz HC. Patient activity, sports participation, and impact loading on the durability of cemented total hip replacements. Clin Orthop 1991; 269:25–31.

[30] D'Souza SR, Sadiq S, New AM, Northmore-Ball MD. Proximal femoral osteotomy as the primary operation for young adults who have osteoarthrosis of the hip. J Bone Joint Surg Am 1998;80(10):1428–38.

[31] Siebenrock KA, Schoeniger R, Ganz R. Anterior femoro-acetabular impingement due to acetabular retroversion. Treatment with periacetabular osteotomy. J Bone Joint Surg Am 2003; 85-A(2):278–86.

[32] Millis MB, Kim YJ. Rationale of osteotomy and related procedures for hip preservation: a review. Clin Orthop 2002;405:108–21.

[33] Fleisig GS, Andrews JR, Dillman CJ, Escamilla RF. Kinetics of baseball pitching with implications about injury mechanisms. Am J Sports Med 1995;23(2):233–9.

[34] Gore RM, Rogers LF, Bowerman J, Suker J, Compere CL. Osseous manifestations of elbow stress associated with sports activities. AJR Am J Roentgenol 1980;134(5):971–7.

[35] Schmitt H, Hansmann HJ, Brocai DR, Loew M. Long term changes of the throwing arm of former elite javelin throwers. Int J Sports Med 2001;22(4):275–9.

[36] Koh JL, Zwahlen BA, Altchek DW. Arthroscopic treatment of posterior elbow impingement. 67th Annual Meeting, American Academy of Orthopaedic Surgery, Orlando (FL); March, 2000.

[37] Conway J. Thrower's view of the elbow. Professional Baseball Team Physicians' Meeting, Dallas; December, 2002.

[38] Oka Y. Debridement for osteoarthritis of the elbow in athletes. Int Orthop 1999;23(2):91–4.

[39] Andrews JR, Timmerman LA. Outcome of elbow surgery in professional baseball players. Am J Sports Med 1995;23(4):p407–13.

[40] Ogilvie-Harris DJ, Gordon R, MacKay M. Arthroscopic treatment for posterior impingement in degenerative arthritis of the elbow. Arthroscopy 1995;11(4):437–43.

[41] O'Driscoll SW. Operative treatment of elbow arthritis. Curr Opin Rheumatol 1995;7(2):103–6.

[42] Moskal MJ. Arthroscopic treatment of posterior impingement of the elbow in athletes. Clin Sports Med 2001;20(1):11–24.

[43] Rettig AC, Ryan RO, Stone JA. Epidemiology of hand injuries in sports. In: Strickland JW, Rettig AC, editors. Hand injuries in athletes. Philadelphia: WB Saunders; 1992. p. 37–42.

[44] Jones WA. Beware of the sprained wrist: incidence of scapholunate instability. J Bone Joint Surg 1988;70B:293–7.

[45] Mayfield JK, Johnson RP, Kilcoyne RK. Carpal dislocations: pathomechanics and progressive perilunar instability. J Hand Surg 1980;5A:226–41.

[46] Dobyns JH, Linscheid RL, Chao EYS, et al. Traumatic instability of the wrist. In: American Academy of Orthopaedic Surgeons Instructional Course Lectures. St. Louis: CV Mosby; 1975. p. 182–99.

[47] Linscheid RL, Dobyns JH, Beabout JW, et al. Traumatic instability of the wrist. J Bone Joint Surg 1972;54A:1612–32.

[48] Burgess RC. The effect of rotary subluxation of the scaphoid on radioscaphoid contact. J Hand Surg 1987;12A:771–4.

[49] Cohen MS. Ligamentous injuries of the wrist in the athlete. Clin Sports Med 1998;17:533–51.

[50] Rettig AC, Patel DV. Epidemiology of elbow, forearm and wrist injuries in the athlete. Clin Sports Med 1995;31:289–97.

[51] Riester JN, Baker BE, Mosher JF, et al. A review of scaphoid fracture healing in competitive athletes. Am J Sports Med 1985;13:159–61.

[52] Panagis JS, Gelberman JH, Taleisnik J, et al. The arterial anatomy of the human carpus. Part II: the intraosseous vascularity. J Hand Surg 1983;8A:375–82.

[53] Mack GR, Bosse MJ, Gelberman RH, et al. The natural history of scaphoid non-union. J Bone Joint Surg 1984;66A:504–9.

[54] Ruby LK, Stinson J, Belsky MR. The natural history of scaphoid non-union: a review of 55 cases. J Bone Joint Surg 1985;67A:428–32.

[55] Bradway JK, Amadio PC, Cooney WP. Open reduction and internal fixation of displaced, comminuted intra-articular fractures of the distal radius. J Bone Joint Surg 1989;71A:839–47.

[56] Knirk JL, Jupiter JB. Intraarticular fractures of the distal end of the radius in young adults. J Bone Joint Surg Am 1986;68:647–59.

[57] Catalano LW, Cole RJ, Gelberman RH, Evanoff BA, Gilula LA, Borrelli J. Displaced intra-articular fractures of the distal aspect of the radius. long term results in young adults after open reduction internal fixation. J Bone Joint Surg Am 1997;79:1290–302.

[58] Rettig AC. Athletic injuries of the wrist and hand. Am J Sports Med 2003;31:1038–48.

[59] Buckner JD. Acute dislocations of the distal radioulnar joint. J Bone Joint Surg 1995;77A: 958–68.

[60] Watson HK, Ryu JY, Burgess RC. Matched distal ulnar resection. J Hand Surg Am 1986;11: 812–7.

[61] Coyle MP, Carroll RE. Dysfunction of the pistriquestral joint: treatment by pisiform excision. J Hand Surg Am 1982;7:421.

[62] Jenkins SA. Osteoarthritis of the piso-triquetral joint: report of three cases. J Bone Joint Surg Br 1951;33B:532.

[63] McMurray TP. Footballers ankle. J Bone Joint Surg 1950;32-B:68.

[64] Parkes 2nd JC, Hamilton WG, Patterson AH, Rawles Jr JG. The anterior impingement syndrome of the ankle. J Trauma 1980;20(10):895–8.

[65] Schmitt H, Lemke JM, Brocai DR, Parsch D. Degenerative changes in the ankle in former elite high jumpers. Clin J Sport Med 2003;13(1):6–10.

[66] Scranton Jr PE, McDermott JE. Anterior tibial spurs: a comparison of open versus arthroscopic debridement. Foot Ankle 1992;13:125–9.

[67] Reynaert P, Gelen G, Geens G. Arthroscopic treatment of anterior impingement of the ankle. Acta Orthop Belg 1994;60(4):p384–8.

[68] van Dijk CN, Tol JL, Verheyen CC. A prospective study of prognostic factors concerning the outcome of arthroscopic surgery for anterior ankle impingement. Am J Sports Med 1997; 25(6):737–45.

[69] Philbin TM, Lee TH, Berlet GC. Arthroscopy for athletic foot and ankle injuries. Clin Sports Med 2004;23:1.

[70] Coester LM, Saltzman CL, Leupold J, Pontarelli W. Long-term results following ankle arthrodesis for post-traumatic arthritis. J Bone Joint Surg Am 2001;83-A(2):219–28.

[71] Knecht SI, Estin M, Callaghan JJ, Zimmerman MB, Alliman KJ, Alvine FG, et al. The agility total ankle arthroplasty. Seven to sixteen-year follow-up. J Bone Joint Surg Am 2004;86-A(6): 1161–71.

[72] Shankar NS. Silastic single-stem implants in the treatment of hallux rigidus. Foot Ankle Int 1995;16:487–91.

[73] Bowers Jr KD, Martin RB. Turf toe: a shoe related football injury. Med Sci Sports Exerc 1976;8:81–3.

[74] Joseph J. Range of movement of the great toe in men. J Bone Joint Surg 1954;36-B:450–7.

[75] Mulier T, Steenwerckx A, Thienport E, Sioen W, Hoore K, Peeraer L, et al. Results after cheilectomy in athletes with hallux rigidus. Foot Ankle Int 1999;20:232–7.

ELSEVIER
SAUNDERS

Clin Sports Med 24 (2005) 71–82

CLINICS
IN SPORTS
MEDICINE

The Use of NSAIDs and Nutritional Supplements in Athletes with Osteoarthritis: Prevalence, Benefits, and Consequences

Robert T. Gorsline, MD, Christopher C. Kaeding, MD*

Department of Orthopaedics, The Ohio State University Medical Center, 2050 Kenny Road, Columbus, OH 43221-3502, USA

Participation in sports activities is associated with significant improvements in overall physical and mental health for both young and old. The relative risk for the development of coronary artery disease, diabetes, and hypertension is significantly reduced in patients who engage in regular exercise [1–3]. Although the health benefits of regular exercise are evident, the consequences of physical activity are as yet to be defined.

Physical activity subjects the athlete to physical stresses that may have negative long-term effects. A growing number of studies demonstrate that increased physical activity may be associated with the development of degenerative changes to articular cartilage [4]. Additionally, acute injury can cause posttraumatic arthritis, which may compound the day-to-day stresses of training and physical exertion.

Acute injury and chronic arthritic conditions are common factors that bring both elite and recreational athletes to a physician's office. These individuals present with pain and disability, and have typically started some form of treatment before the office visit. This may be in the form of activity modification, cryotherapy, or bracing; but commonly includes over-the-counter (OTC) medications such as NSAIDs, or nutritional supplements such as glucosamine and chondroitin.

The purpose of this article is to review both acute and chronic sports injury, including osteoarthritis, that result in the use of NSAIDs and nutritional

---

* Corresponding author.
  E-mail address: Kaeding-1@medctr.osu.edu (C.C. Kaeding).

sportsmed.theclinics.com

supplements. The behavior of NSAID and supplement use will be explored, as well as the side effect profiles of these drugs.

Sports injuries and osteoarthritis

If one includes both acute injury and the exposure to stresses that may lead to chronic injury and degenerative joint disease; physical activity represents a major risk factor for injury [4]. Not only does injury affect the patient with regard to disability and reduced quality of life, but sports injury burdens society with the cost of treatment, and time lost from work.

Numerous studies have attempted to quantify the incidence of injury. These studies are limited, however, due to the variety of sports that are played and the exposure level of each activity. In addition to the variety of physical activities that individuals participate in, a significant variation exists in the individuals themselves. Height, weight, genetics, and gender are but a few confounding variables that make the incidence of sport injury difficult to interpret.

Although certainly not inclusive of the entire spectrum of athletes and individuals participating in physical activities, several cohort studies have been performed that provide some information as to the relative rate of injury in physically active persons.

In a prospective study of 324 Irish athletes over a 1-year period, Watson et al determined that the average incidence of acute injury per year was 1.17, and for overuse injuries was 0.93. This data represented athletes who competed at a county level, in club sports at a national level, and at an international level. The activities included, running, hurling, football, gymnastics, basketball, rowing, and tennis. Dividing the activities into endurance, contact, and noncontact sports yielded the following incidence of injury: for acute injury the rates were 1.17, 0.996, and 1.580 per year, respectively, and for overuse injury the rates were 1.061, 0.766, and 1.136 per year, respectively [5].

Another prospective study of 265 intercollegiate football players concluded that the probability of injury was 106.7% for 5 years, 99.1% for 4 years, and 46.6% for 1 year. The data analyzed was from daily injury and illness reports, and included musculoskeletal complaints as well as ophthalmologic problems, heat-related problems, and upper respiratory and gastrointestinal infections. The most common musculoskeletal injuries were knee and ankle injuries [6]. This study was limited with respect to the population: an all male athlete participating in a contact sport.

Looking at female athletes, Engstrom et al analyzed injuries in a prospective study of elite soccer players. During a 1-year period, medical students registered all injuries to 41 players on two female teams during training and competition. The incidence of injury was 24/1000 hours of competitive play and 7/1000 hours of training. Eighty-eight percent of the injuries were to the lower extremity, 72% were acute injuries, while 28% were overuse injuries. Eight percent of the players suffered some form of injury during the year [7].

Although these groups vary with regard to gender and sport played, they represent a group of athletes who engage in strenuous physical activity on a daily basis. Combining theses studies, one could estimate the incidence of injury in these athletes for both acute and chronic injury to approach one injury per year. These studies have limitations in that they are not applicable to the patients who engage in sports as a whole. To formulate an incidence of injury for all physically active patients that accounts for the variables of activity, intensity of training, gender, age, weight, genetic makeup, and so on, is an impossible task. Additionally, although these studies give insight into the incidence of injuries that occur in athletic populations, they do not address the long-term consequence of injury in this population. To what degree do the stresses of daily exercise contribute to the formation of osteoarthritis? Do acute injuries contribute to the development of degenerative changes in the joints? Variability in joint shape, joint stability, and the genetics of cartilage response to injury, all contribute to the difficulty in interpreting any one study [8]. Despite these limitations, there are emerging studies indicating that physical activity is a risk factor for the development of osteoarthritis.

For example, Kujala et al performed a retrospective review on former elite male athletes. Using a registry of Finnish male athletes who competed at an Olympic or other international level between 1920 and 1965, the study looked at relative risks of development of chronic disease. Although the participants had significant improvement in health with respect to coronary artery disease, diabetes, and hypertension, an increase in the development of osteoarthritis was noted in these athletes. The cohort was divided into endurance sports (runners and crosscountry skiers), mixed sports (soccer, basketball, and ice hockey), and power sports (boxing, wrestling, and weight lifting). The relative risks for osteoarthritis were 2.42, 2.37, and 2.68, respectively [3].

In a retrospective study, Spector et al evaluated 81 female ex-elite middle long-distance runners and tennis players. In comparison to 997 age-matched controls, the athletes demonstrated a relative risk of 2.5 for hip arthritis, and 3.5 for knee arthritis [9]. A cross-sectional study performed by Lindberg et al demonstrated a 5.8% incidence of hip osteoarthritis in 286 ex-soccer players compared with a 2.8% incidence in controls [10].

Contradicting this information are studies in long-distance runners, which fail to demonstrate an increased risk for osteoarthritis. Lane et al retrospectively studied 41 long-distance runners averaging 5 hours per week of running over 9 years, concluding that there was no increased risk of osteoarthritis in runners [11]. Konradsen et al evaluated 58 ex-long-distance runners who averaged >20 km per week of running over 40 years and compared them to age, weight, and occupation-matched controls. Radiographically, the athletic cohort had no significant changes suggestive of osteoarthritis when compared with controls [12].

Although it is not a consensus opinion of these articles, excessive microtrauma from exercise can potentially increase the risk of developing osteoarthritis. This risk is dependent on the amount, type, and intensity of the exercise, as well as the genetics, joint structure, fitness, and body habitus of the individual [13]. Also, acute injury to joints, to which athletes are at increased risk, can increase the risk of developing osteoarthritis. This is particularly true if these athletes have ligament instability or have undergone a complete or partial meniscectomy for a meniscal tear [4,14].

Antiinflammatory treatment of sport injury and osteoarthritis

The development of NSAIDs progressed significantly in the twentieth century, becoming one of the largest classes of drugs in the pharmaceutical industry. The landmark discovery by Sir John Vane in 1971, that aspirin's mechanism of action was the inhibition of cyclooxygenase (COX), an enzyme that converts arachadonic acid into prostaglandins, led to the characterization of the pathophysiology of inflammation and the development of these novel antiinflammatory drugs [15]. There are now large volumes of literature regarding the inflammatory and pain mediating effects of arachadonic acid derivatives [15–17].

Arachadonic acid is a 20-carbon fatty acid molecule that exists in numerous cell types bound to the membrane lipids phospatidylcholine or phosphatidylinositol. It is cleaved from its membrane bound form by the action of intra cellular phospholipases. Once released, arachadonic acid is rapidly metabolized along two pathways into potent mediators of inflammation. (1) It is metabolized by COX into prostaglandins (PGD_2, PGE_2, PGF_2, and PGI_2) and thromboxanes (TxA_2). (2) It is metabolized by lipoxygenase (LOX) into leukotrienes (LTB_4, LTC_4, LTD_4, and LTE_4). This metabolic pathway is the target for drugs that inhibit inflammation. The site of action of NSAIDs is the competitive inhibition of COX, while the steroid-based antiinflammatory drugs inhibit arachadonic acid release and the transcription of the COX gene [18].

Further advancement in the NSAID industry occurred in the early 1990s with the discovery of two isoforms of the COX gene. Prompted by a need for NSAIDs with fewer gastrointestinal and renal side effects, industry research yielded the discovery of an inducible form of COX that is expressed during injury and promotes inflammation. The current understanding of the function of the COX isoforms are as follows: COX-1 functions in physiologic maintenance by producing prostaglandins critical for normal renal function, gastric mucosal integrity, and hemostasis [19]. High concentrations of COX-1 are found in platelets, vascular endothelial cells, gastric cells, and in kidney collecting tubules. COX-2 is undetectable in physiologic conditions and inflammatory mediators including interleukin-1, tumor necrosis factor, and lipopolysaccharide induce its expression up to 80-fold. Furthermore, COX-2 can be selectively inhibited, leading to lower gastrointestinal and renal side effects [19,20].

NSAID efficacy in the treatment of osteoarthritis has been extensively studied. In two large meta-analyses, 14 out of 14 studies of hip osteoarthritis, and 8 out of 9 studies of knee osteoarthritis, demonstrated increased efficacy of NSAIDs compared with placebo [21,22]. This data showed almost equal efficacy for traditional NSAIDs. The COX-2 selective NSAIDs have fewer studies regarding their efficacy, but appear to be as effective. Simon et al performed a study on 293 patients with a new onset flare of knee osteoarthritis, and concluded that Celecoxib provided significantly greater pain relief that placebo [22,23]. In addition, Cannon et al performed a prospective study on patients with hip and knee osteoarthritis and randomized them to Rofecoxib or Diclofenac. This study demonstrated equal efficacy between selective COX-2 and traditional NSAIDs [24].

There is strong evidence that NSAIDs provide significant relief from the pain and inflammation associated with osteoarthritis. Unfortunately, the literature is not as clear regarding the role of NSAIDs in both acute and chronic soft tissue injury.

Nutritional supplements in the treatment of osteoarthritis

The publication of "The Arthritis Cure" in 1997 by Theodosakis and colleagues initiated one of the most controversial debates in current medicine [25]. Following publication of this book, there was an explosion of interest in glucosamine as a treatment for osteoarthritis. Anecdotal reports emerged as to the benefits of glucosamine, and contentions were made that traditional medicine was overlooking a safe and simple treatment in favor of products developed by the pharmaceutical industry [26]. The lack of a pharmacologic mechanism, limited studies published in obscure journals, as well as questionable scientific methodology of the available studies, contributed to the skepticism of the scientific community [22,26]. Since the initial publications, however, there have been large meta-analysis, as well as tissue culture and animal model data, that supports the benefit of glucosamine in osteoarthritis [27]. Chondroitin, similarly, has had growing support, both in clinical trials and in animal studies, for its use in arthritis. Controversy over efficacy notwithstanding, glucosamine and chondroitin are widely used nutraceuticals that have a growing OTC use.

Glucosamine sulfate is a primary building block of proteoglycans, and is present in hyaline cartilage. Oral administration of glucosamine leads to a rapid degradation and near complete gastrointestinal absorption. Following absorption, there is a substantial first-pass hepatic metabolism [28]. Based on radioactive labeling studies, glucosamine is widely distributed throughout the body, and includes the joints [29,30]. In vitro studies have determined that glucosamine inhibits interleukin-1 induced nitric oxide production and has a modest anti-inflammatory effect in the rat [30]. Early clinical studies included placebo-controlled randomized studies that were limited by small size, short duration of treatment, and nonvalidated outcomes measures. More recently, there have been several meta-analyses that provide some more substantiated scientific methodology to the assessment of glucosamine.

McAlindon and colleagues performed a meta-analyses that included published and unpublished randomized, double-blinded, placebo-controlled trials of glucosamine for treatment of symptomatic hip and knee osteoarthritis [31]. The analysis included quality assessment of each article and validated assessment measurements. The conclusions were that collectively, glucosamine demonstrated efficacy in the treatment of osteoarthritis; however, the efficacy was likely exaggerated due to publication bias and methodology of the various trials [26].

Towheed et al also performed a meta-analysis of 16 randomized controlled clinical trials of glucosamine as a treatment of osteoarthritis [32]. Overall, glucosamine was found to be safe and effective for the treatment of osteoarthritis. In 13 of the studies where glucosamine was compared with placebo, 12 studies demonstrated superior pain relief for glucosamine. In four studies that compared glucosamine to NSAIDs, two studies demonstrated improved efficacy for glucosamine and two showed NSAIDs to be superior [33].

More recently, Hughes and Carr published a prospective, placebo-controlled, double-blind, randomized study of glucosamine in osteoarthritis of the knee [34]. This study included 80 participants randomized to glucosamine sulfate 500 mg three times a day, or placebo. Unlike previous studies, this study had sound methodology, was independent of industrial sponsors, and had a clear analytic approach [26]. The results were less favorable, with no significant difference between groups.

Similar in controversy is the supplement chondroitin sulfate. Predominately derived from beef trachea, chondroitin sulfate is a large molecule that has a limited bioavailability of 15% from an oral dose. It is distributed throughout the body, and with radioactive labeling studies has been shown to reach joint tissues. The theoretic physiologic effects of chondroitin are that it stimulates proteoglycan synthesis, inhibits proteoglycan degradation, and enhances the production of hyaluronic acid [28]. Bassleer et al demonstrated that chondrocytes treated with chondroitin could be stimulated to replace or repair damaged proteoglycans [35]. Additionally, chondroitin appears to have modest antiinflammatory and metabolic effects on chondrocytes [30]. Although clinical studies are limited, there is data demonstrating a reduction in the use of NSAIDs in osteoarthritis patients who use oral chondroitin sulfate [28,36].

There are multiple products on the marketplace that are labeled as chondroitin and glucosamine, and this introduces further difficulties in assessing the benefit of these nutraceuticals. Adebowale et al analyzed the content of several marketplace products and determined that the amount of glucosamine and chondroitin varied significantly from the labeled amount on the package [33,37].

Further confusing conclusions regarding the efficacy of glucosamine and chondroitin is the universal acceptance of nutraceuticals by the veterinary community for the treatment of lameness. A survey of 2524 veterinarians using both glucosamine sulfate and chondroitin sulfate had the following results: The most common animal treated was the dog; however, 47% of respondents used the drug on other animals. The clinical efficacy of nutraceuticals were deemed good or excellent in alleviating pain by 83% of respondents, and for improving mobility it was rated good or excellent by 89% of respondents [27,38]. In addition, Hanson et al performed a double-blind, placebo-controlled, randomized study in horses. The outcomes measured were lameness, overall clinical condition, and owner assessment. Significant improvements were reported in each group for glucosamine and chondroitin when compared with placebo [27,39].

There is still much controversy in the literature regarding the clinical efficacy of nutraceuticals such as glucosamine and chondroitin. In an effort to make clear the efficacy and toxicity of these drugs, the National Institutes of Health is currently performing a large-scale multicenter controlled study.

Side effects of NSAIDs and nutritional supplements

The primary adverse effects of NSAIDs involve the gastrointestinal system, renal system, and coagulation system. These side effects can result from single-dose administration or chronic use, and are related to the inhibition of normal prostaglandin function. The most common adverse effects are gastrointestinal complaints, which range in severity from dyspepsia to gastric perforation and bleeding. The adverse effects of traditional NSAIDs will be reviewed by organ system, followed by a summary of adverse reactions to COX-2 selective agents.

The ability of the NSAIDs to induce gastrointestinal mucosal damage is well described [40,41]. It is estimated that gastrointestinal (GI) bleeding and perforation related to NSAIDs are responsible for 200,000 to 400,000 hospitalizations each year in the United States [18]. The rates of gastroduodenal ulceration confirmed by endoscopy have been placed at 15% to 30% [22]. These studies are related to chronic use of NSAIDs, but there are certainly risks associated with OTC use of NSAIDs. Lanza et al studied patients with a 1- to 10-day history of NSAIDs use. They used endoscopy to rate the GI mucousa of the subjects from 0 to 4 (0—normal mucousa, 4—superficial ulceration) and evaluated several OTC pain relievers. The results were as follows: Ibuprofen (1200 mg/d) 0.46, enteric-coated Aspirin (3900 mg/d) 0.84, Aspirin (2600 mg/d) 3.07, and Naproxen (500 mg/d) 1.17 [40,42]. Clearly, even the use of NSAIDs within OTC guidelines is associated with gastrointestinal side effects. Risk factors for GI complications include: age > 65, history of ulcer disease, smoking, alcohol use, and concomitant corticosteroid use. Strategies to reduce the GI side effects of traditional NSAIDs have included the parallel use of histamine$_2$ receptor antagonists, proton pump inhibitors, and prostaglandin analogs. These strategies are successful in the reduction of gastric mucosal damage; however, they are not ideal.

The renal side effects of NSAIDs are more difficult to define. One study estimates the rate of serious renal problems requiring hospitalization at between 0.5% and 1% for chronic NSAID users. Additionally, a retrospective review of patients using NSAIDs for the treatment of rheumatoid arthritis demonstrated a significant elevation in serum creatinine in 3.8% of patients who used Ibuprofen, and in 5.7% of patients who used Aspirin. However, none of theses laboratory changes were noted to have clinical consequences [40]. Apparently, the healthy kidney has the ability to compensate for prostaglandin inhibition; however, when baseline renal function is impaired, renal function suffers. The risk factors associated with serious renal sequelae from NSAIDs are: age >65, hypertension, dehydration, and concomitant use of diuretics and ACE inhibitors [22,40,43].

Platelet dysfunction is universally recognized with regard to NSAIDs. The mild systemic antiplatelet effect is caused by inhibition of thromboxane A_2 production. Spontaneous bleeding complications outside the gastrointestinal tract very rarely result from the use of aspirin and other NSAIDs in individuals who are otherwise hemostatically normal. Most surgical procedures are not usually associated with clinically significant bleeding in patients taking these drugs, making it typically unnecessary to discontinue them and thus delay surgery for the purpose of restoring normal hemostasis. Factors that increase the risk of bleeding with aspirin and other NSAIDs include: coexisting coagulation abnormalities, alcohol use, and the simultaneous use of anticoagulants [44].

The COX-2 selective NSAIDs show less inhibition of physiologic prostaglandin production; however, they all have some degree of COX-1 suppression, and therefore have adverse effects. GI bleeding is significantly lower in the COX-2 selective agents compared with traditional NSAIDs. Short-term endoscopic studies suggest that Celecoxib at therapeutic doses has minimal effect on gastric mucousa. Similarly, Rofecoxib has been shown to have a significantly lower incidence of gastroduodenal ulcers in endoscopic studies [19]. In addition, studies demonstrate that Celecoxib has minimal antiplatelet activity at both therapeutic and supratherapeutic doses [45]. Although the rate of adverse effects of COX-2 selective NSAIDs is not zero, it is significantly less than that associated with traditional NSAIDs.

The side effects of glucosamine and chondroitin are not as clearly defined as those of NSAIDs. In a large study of glucosamine, only 14 patients out of 1000 were withdrawn due to side effects [32]. For both glucosamine and chondroitin, the most common complaints from patients are related to the GI tract, and occur with similar frequency of placebo [30]. There is some evidence that glucosamine may interfere with glucose homeostasis. Chan and colleagues have demonstrated evidence that glucosamine may increase insulin resistance. They recommend glucose monitoring in patients on long-term therapy [33]. The overall side effect profile of both glucosamine and chondroitin currently appears to be equal to placebo. This conclusion is drawn from a variety of randomized controlled studies as well as from large meta-analyses [31,33].

Behavioral aspects of NSAID and nutraceutical use

OTC and nonprescription medication use is highly prevalent in society, with studies demonstrating 30% of adults having used nonprescription medication in the previous 48 hours [46]. In 1993, more than $2.7 billion was spend on OTC analgesics, with a reported 50 million Americans using NSAIDs [43]. More recent data places these figures at 13 million Americans using NSAIDs daily, and world wide sales totaling $5.7 billion [19]. Glucosamine and chondroitin are widely used as well. Together, these products rank as the third best-selling nutraceuticals, with sales in the United States totaling $369 million. It has been estimated that 5% to 8% of the adults in the United States have at one point in time used glucosamine or chondroitin [26].

The widespread use of these drugs is readily evident, but what are the attitudes of the individual using them? Are the products used according to the package recommendations? What are the perceptions of patients with respect to safety and recommended doses? These questions are difficult to answer due to the limited literature on this subject. There are no studies on attitudes and behaviors related to glucosamine and chondroitin use, and there are limited studies related to NSAIDs.

Warner et al performed a study on adolescent male athletes to better understand behavior of NSAID use [46]. In this study, 681 self-administered questionnaires were obtained from high school football players. The questionnaire included information on sociodemographics, perceived advantages and disadvantages of NSAIDs, as well as perceptions regarding improved performance. Seventy-five percent of respondents had used NSAIDs within the last 3 months for reasons related to their sport. Fifteen percent used NSAIDs on a daily basis. Thirty-eight percent of the respondents administered the medication independent of an adult, and 29% of them dosed the medication independent of adult supervision. The overall conclusions of the study were that NSAID use in the group was prevalent, recognition of disadvantages (side effects) low, and despite package inserts recommending against chronic use, one in seven athletes used NSAIDs daily for prolonged periods of time.

This data was compiled from a population that was adolescent, 90% white, and 88% privately insured. It certainly does not represent the population as a whole, but it points out the possibilities of some alarming problems. NSAIDs may not necessarily be used according to the recommendations of the package. They may be used on a daily basis for a long period of time. The possible side effects may not be apparent compared with the perceived advantages gained by decreased pain and increased performance. This type of behavior and attitude may be prevalent in athletic populations regardless of age and level of competition.

The use of NSAIDs by printed OTC guidelines, and the use of glucosamine and chondroitin, which have no such guidelines, are associated with a calculable level of adverse effects. This, however, may have limited application to the individual who misuses these drugs. The athlete who is subjected to intermittent dehydration and uses OTC NSAIDs daily may have a much higher rate of renal problems than can be currently estimated. To better advise patients on risks associated with OTC medication, a better understanding is needed on the behaviors and attitudes related to the use of these products.

Summary

Athletes represent a subset of the population that is at risk for the development of chronic overuse syndromes and osteoarthritis. This risk is related to a variety of factors including, but not limited to: age, previous injury, genetics, and type, frequency, and intensity of activity. Depending on the severity of the injury, the athlete will potentially initiate treatment with activity modification, cryotherapy, and OTC medications. Additionally, athletes may use nutraceuticals to reduce dependence on NSAIDs to control pain and discomfort. These patients have the potential of presenting to the physician already using drugs to alleviate symptoms. It the responsibility of the treating physician to discuss the use of OTC medications and nutraceutical use as well as to ensure that these medications are used appropriately.

References

[1] Kohl 3rd HW. Physical activity and cardiovascular disease: evidence for a dose response. Med Sci Sports Exerc 2001;33(6):S472–83, S93–4.

[2] Kelley DE, Goodpaster BH. Effects of exercise on glucose homeostasis in Type 2 diabetes mellitus. Med Sci Sports Exerc 2001;33(6):S28–9.

[3] Kujala UM, Marti P, Kaprio J, Hernelahti M, Tikkanen H, Sarna S. Occurrence of chronic disease in former top-level athletes. Predominance of benefits, risks or selection effects? Sports Med 2003;33(8):553–61.

[4] Saxon L, Finch C, Bass S. Sports participation, sports injuries and osteoarthritis: implications for prevention. Sports Med 1999;28(2):123–35.

[5] Watson AW. Incidence and nature of sports injuries in Ireland. Analysis of four types of sport. Am J Sports Med 1993;21(1):137–43.

[6] Canale ST, Cantler Jr ED, Sisk TD, Freeman III BL. A chronicle of injuries of an American intercollegiate football team. Am J Sports Med 1981;9(6):384–9.

[7] Engstrom B, Johansson C, Tornkvist H. Soccer injuries among elite female players. Am J Sports Med 1991;19(4):372–5.

[8] Lane NE, Buckwalter JA. Exercise: a cause of osteoarthritis? Rheum Dis Clin North Am 1993;19(3):617–33.

[9] Spector TD, Harris PA, Hart DJ, Cicuttini FM, Nandra D, Etherington J, et al. Risk of osteo-arthritis associated with long-term weight-bearing sports: a radiologic survey of the hips and knees in female ex-athletes and population controls. Arthritis Rheum 1996;39(6):988–95.

[10] Lindberg H, Roos H, Gardsell P. Prevalence of coxarthrosis in former soccer players. 286 players compared with matched controls. Acta Orthop Scand 1993;64(2):165–7.

[11] Lane NE, Bloch DA, Jones HH, Marshall Jr WH, Wood PD, Fries JF. Long-distance running, bone density, and osteoarthritis. JAMA 1986;255(9):1147–51.

[12] Konradsen L, Hansen EM, Sondergaard L. Long distance running and osteoarthrosis. Am J Sports Med 1990;18(4):379–81.

[13] Buckwalter JA, Lane NE. Athletics and osteoarthritis. Am J Sports Med 1997;25(6):873–81.

[14] Rangger C, Kathrein A, Klestil T, Glotzer W. Partial meniscectomy and osteoarthritis. Implications for treatment of athletes. Sports Med 1997;23(1):61–8.

[15] Stanley KL, Weaver JE. Pharmacologic management of pain and inflammation in athletes. Clin Sports Med 1998;17(2):375–92.

[16] Vane JR, Botting RM. Anti-inflammatory drugs and their mechanism of action. Inflamm Res 1998;47(Suppl 2):S78–87.

[17] Abramson S, Weissmann G. The mechanisms of action of nonsteroidal antiinflammatory drugs. Clin Exp Rheumatol 1989;7(Suppl 3):S163–70.

[18] Vance DE, Vance JE. Biochemistry of lipids, lipoproteins, and membranes, Vol. xxi. Amsterdam: Elsevier; 1991. p. 297–326.

[19] Kaplan-Machlis B, Klostermeyer BS. The cyclooxygenase-2 inhibitors: safety and effectiveness. Ann Pharmacother 1999;33(9):979–88.

[20] Siegle I, Klein T, Backman JT, Saal JG, Nusing RM, Fritz P. Expression of cyclooxygenase 1 and cyclooxygenase 2 in human synovial tissue: differential elevation of cyclooxygenase 2 in inflammatory joint diseases. Arthritis Rheum 1998;41(1):122–9.

[21] Towheed TE, Hochberg MC. A systematic review of randomized controlled trials of pharmacological therapy in osteoarthritis of the hip. J Rheumatol 1997;24(2):349–57.

[22] Goldberg SH, Von Feldt JM, Lonner JH. Pharmacologic therapy for osteoarthritis. Am J Orthop 2002;31(12):673–80.

[23] Simon LS, Lanza FL, Lipsky PE, Hubbard RC, Talwalker S, Schwartz BD, et al. Preliminary study of the safety and efficacy of SC-58635, a novel cyclooxygenase 2 inhibitor: efficacy and safety in two placebo-controlled trials in osteoarthritis and rheumatoid arthritis, and studies of gastrointestinal and platelet effects. Arthritis Rheum 1998;41(9):1591–602.

[24] Cannon GW, Caldwell JR, Holt P, McLean B, Seidenberg B, Bolognese J, et al. Rofecoxib, a specific inhibitor of cyclooxygenase 2, with clinical efficacy comparable with that of diclofenac sodium: results of a one-year, randomized, clinical trial in patients with osteoarthritis of the knee and hip. Rofecoxib Phase III Protocol 035 Study Group. Arthritis Rheum 2000;43(5): 978–87.

[25] Theodosakis J, Adderly B, Fox B. 1st edition. The arthritis cure: the medical miracle that can halt, reverse, and may even cure osteoarthritis, vol. xvi. New York: St. Martin's Press; 1997.

[26] McAlindon T. Why are clinical trials of glucosamine no longer uniformly positive? Rheum Dis Clin North Am 2003;29(4):789–801.

[27] Hungerford DS, Jones LC. Glucosamine and chondroitin sulfate are effective in the management of osteoarthritis. J Arthroplasty 2003;18(3):5–9.

[28] Schwenk TL, Costley CD. When food becomes a drug: nonanabolic nutritional supplement use in athletes. Am J Sports Med 2002;30(6):907–16.

[29] Setnikar I, Giacchetti C, Zanolo G. Pharmacokinetics of glucosamine in the dog and in man. Arzneimittelforschung 1986;36(4):729–35.

[30] Felson DT, McAlindon TE. Glucosamine and chondroitin for osteoarthritis: to recommend or not to recommend? Arthritis Care Res 2000;13(4):179–82.

[31] McAlindon TE, LaValley MP, Gulin JP, Felson DT. Glucosamine and chondroitin for treatment of osteoarthritis: a systematic quality assessment and meta-analysis. JAMA 2000;283(11): 1469–75.

[32] Towheed TE, Anastassiades TP, Shea B, Houpt J, Welch V, Hochberg MC. Glucosamine therapy for treating osteoarthritis. Cochrane Database Syst Rev 2001;1:CD002946.

[33] Towheed TE. Current status of glucosamine therapy in osteoarthritis. Arthritis Rheum 2003; 49(4):601–4.

[34] Hughes R, Carr A. A randomized, double-blind, placebo-controlled trial of glucosamine sulphate as an analgesic in osteoarthritis of the knee. Rheumatology (Oxford) 2002;41(3):279–84.

[35] Bassleer C, Henrotin Y, Franchimont P. In-vitro evaluation of drugs proposed as chondroprotective agents. Int J Tissue React 1992;14(5):231–41.

[36] Uebelhart D, Thonar EJ, Delmas PD, Chantraine A, Vignon E. Effects of oral chondroitin sulfate on the progression of knee osteoarthritis: a pilot study. Osteoarthritis Cartilage 1998;6(Suppl A): 39–46.

[37] Adebowale A, Cox D, Liang Z, Eddington N. Analysis of glucosamine and chondroitin sulfate content in marketed products and the caco-2 permeability of chondroitin sulfate raw materials. J Am Nutraceut Assoc 2000;3:37–44.

[38] Anderson MA, Slater MR, Hammad TA. Results of a survey of small-animal practitioners on the perceived clinical efficacy and safety of an oral nutraceutical. Prev Vet Med 1999;38(1): 65–73.

[39] Hansen R, Brawner W, Blaik M. Oral treatment with a nutraceutical (Cosequin) for ameliorating signs of navicular syndrome in horses. Vet Ther 2001;2:148–59.
[40] Hersh EV, Moore PA, Ross GL. Over-the-counter analgesics and antipyretics: a critical assessment. Clin Ther 2000;22(5):500–48.
[41] Langman MJ, Weil J, Wainwright P, Lawson DH, Rawlins MD, Logan RF, et al. Risks of bleeding peptic ulcer associated with individual non-steroidal anti-inflammatory drugs. Lancet 1994;343(8905):1075–8.
[42] Lanza FL. Endoscopic studies of gastric and duodenal injury after the use of ibuprofen, aspirin, and other nonsteroidal anti-inflammatory agents. Am J Med 1984;77(1A):19–24.
[43] Whelton A. Renal effects of over-the-counter analgesics. J Clin Pharmacol 1995;35(5):454–63.
[44] Schafer AI. Effects of nonsteroidal anti-inflammatory therapy on platelets. Am J Med 1999; 106(5B):25S–36S.
[45] Mengle-Gaw L, Hubbard RC, Karim A. A study of the platelet effects of SC-58635, a novel COX-2 selective inhibitor (abstract). Arthritis Rheum 1997;40(Suppl):S93–374A.
[46] Warner DC, Schnepf G, Barrett MS, Dian D, Swigonski NL. Prevalence, attitudes, and behaviors related to the use of nonsteroidal anti-inflammatory drugs (NSAIDs) in student athletes. J Adolesc Health 2002;30(3):150–3.

ELSEVIER
SAUNDERS

CLINICS
IN SPORTS
MEDICINE

Clin Sports Med 24 (2005) 83–91

Use of Injections for Osteoarthritis in Joints and Sports Activity

Jason C. Snibbe, MD*, Ralph A. Gambardella, MD

Kerlan-Jobe Orthopaedic Clinic, 6801 Park Terrace, Los Angeles, CA 90045, USA

Osteoarthritis is the most common form of arthritis, and can be a major source of disability. Traditional nonoperative treatment includes activity modification, weight loss, exercise, assistive devices, nonsteroidal antiinflammatory medications (NSAIDs), analgesics, and corticosteroid injections. Specifically, NSAID treatment is associated with significant morbidity to the gastrointestinal system. The economic burden of the gastrointestinal side effects of NSAIDs is estimated to exceed $500 million annually [1]. Surgical treatment of osteoarthritis of the hip and knee is effective, but not indicated for early stages of the disease in all patients. There are also potential complications and enormous costs associated with surgery.

Since the early 1950s, intraarticular corticosteroids have been widely used to manage arthritic conditions. Hollander et al showed that intraarticular hydrocortisone decreases the leukocyte count and temperature of the synovial fluid [2]. More recent studies have shown superior antiinflammatory effects of tertiary-butyl esters of hydrocortisone compared to hydrocortisone [3]. Intraarticular corticosteroids are accepted as an important treatment modality, but currently there are no guidelines in regard to administration. Even less information is known in regard to intraarticular corticosteroid injections and the treatment of sports injuries.

In recent years, intraarticular viscosupplementation with hyaluronate-derived products has gained popularity as a modality for the treatment of osteoarthritis of the knee. Hyaluronic acid provides the elastic and viscous function of synovial fluid, protecting the joint from compressive and shear forces. The content of synovial fluid, in the presence of osteoarthritis, has a decreased concentration

---

* Corresponding author.
E-mail address: jsnibbe@yahoo.com (J.C. Snibbe).

and molecular weight of hyaluronic acid. This process reduces the viscosity and the protective function of the synovial fluid.

The initial rational for the intraarticular injection of hyaluronic acid was to restore the viscoelasticity of synovial fluid. Several studies have shown that injected hyaluronic acid can augment the flow of synovial fluid, normalize the synthesis and inhibit the degradation of endogenous hyaluronic acid, and relieve joint pain [4,25].

Corticosteroids

Mechanism of action

Corticosteroids are a well-known antiinflammatory, but their mechanism of action is not completely known. Corticosteroids are highly lipid soluble, and bind to receptors in the nuclei of cells. Corticosteroids inhibit the accumulation of inflammatory cells, such as leukocytes and neutrophils. They prevent phagocytosis, lysosomal enzyme release, and the synthesis of several inflammatory mediators.

Recent studies have shown that intraarticular corticosteroid injections decrease neutrophil migration into inflamed joints of patients with osteoarthritis [5]. The authors speculated that the mechanism of action is by blocking the action of macrophage inhibitory factor, which reduces vascular permeability and cell adhesion and migration. In addition, intraarticular corticosteroids reduce prostaglandin synthesis up to 50% and decrease interleukin-1 secretion by the synovium. Intraarticular corticosteroids also inhibit leukocyte secretion from the synovium. This increases the concentration of hyaluronic acid in the joint, which increases the viscosity of the synovial fluid.

Indications

Intraarticular corticosteroid injections are frequently used to treat acute and chronic inflammatory conditions. Injections decrease inflammation and swelling, which decreases pain and increases joint mobility. Results vary, depending on the type of joint injected. Small nonweight-bearing joints have better results that larger weight-bearing joints [3]. The intraarticular corticosteroid cannot prevent the pain derived from weight-bearing forces across the joint. The literature has shown that intraarticular corticosteroid injections for the treatment of osteoarthritis can be variable. Doherty et al, in a double-blind, placebo-controlled study of 59 patients, reported a significant reduction in pain scores 3 weeks after an intraarticular corticosteroid injection [6]. Another comparison of intraarticular triamcinolone and placebo showed greater pain relief with a steroid injection at 1 week, but similar results at later intervals [7]. Intraarticular corticosteroid injections are commonly used for rheumatoid arthritis, and show excellent long-term pain relief. Therefore, it is thought that the primary effect of the corticosteroid is on the synovium. Other indications for intraarticular corticosteroid injections are for adhesive capsulitis of the shoulder. Several studies have shown improved motion up to 6 weeks after injection, but results are short lived and unreliable [3].

There is no clear, objective evidence for intraarticular corticosteroid injections on the treatment of osteoarthritic or sports-related injuries of knees, ankles, shoulders, acromioclavicular joints, lumbar facet joints, and smaller hand and foot joints. Injections around joints are associated with significant risk. Corticosteroid injections around ligaments and tendons inhibit collagen synthesis. Therefore, injections could cause ligament and tendon rupture, which is the reason many orthopedists do not recommend corticosteroid injections in these locations.

The treatment of bursitis and tedonitis, such as the subacromial bursitis, greater trochanteric bursitis, and medial/lateral epicondylitis, are common, and results have varied in the literature. Stahl et al conducted a prospective, randomized, double-blind study on 60 elbows with medial epicondylitis [8]. They reported significant pain relief at 6 weeks after corticosteroid injection. At 3 months, there was no difference in symptoms between the group who had the injection and those who did not. Retrocalcaneal and prepatellar burse injections have less promising efficacy, and are assoiated with tendon rupture. In the presence of inflamed bursae or tendons, the injection of corticosteroids provides some relief, but the duration of relief is usually short lived.

Preparations

Hydrocortisone was the first steroid used for intraarticular injection. Additional research lead to the development of longer lasting compounds in the form of esters of prednisolone, triamcinolone, and dexamethasone. The duration of effect of the corticosteroid is inversely proportional to the solubility.

Table 1
Commonly used corticosteroids

Generic name	Proprietary name	Concentration (mg/mL)	Average duration of effect (days)
Triamcinolone hexacetonide	Aristospan	2	21
Triamcinolone diacetate	Aristocort	25–40	7
Triamcinolone acetonide	Kenalog	10–40	14
Methylprednisolone sodium succinate	Solu-Medrol	40–125	4
Methylprednisolone acetate	Depo-Medrol	40–80	8
Prednisolone tebutate	Hydeltra	20	10–14
Betamethasone acetate	Soluspan	6	9
Dexamethasone acetate	Decadron-LA	8	8
Dexamethasone sodium phosphate	Decadron	4	6
Hydrocortisone acetate	Hydrocortone	25	8

Triamcinolone hexacetonide is the least soluble, and therefore, the longest lasting Table 1 lists the common corticosteroids used in orthopedic treatment (see Table 1).

Contraindications

Suspicion of infection is the main contraindication to intraarticular corticosteroid injection. Active infection of the skin and overlying tissues increases the risk of inoculating the joint during injection. Other absolute contraindications are hypersensitivity, presence of a joint prosthesis, and uncontrolled bleeding diathesis. Relative contraindications include anticoagulation therapy, joint instability, poorly controlled diabetes, and adjacent skin abrasions. Direct injection into a tendon or ligament should always be avoided due to the risk of rupture.

Complications

Adverse effects of corticosteroid injections include local and systemic effects of the medication. The local effects include tendon and ligament rupture, cutaneous atrophy at the injection site, calcification of the joint capsule, and infection. At low doses, the systemic effects are beneficial, which include transient eosinopenia and antiinflammatory effects on distant joints. At higher doses, which occur when treating multiple joints, the corticosteroids can inhibit the hypothalamic–pituitary–adrenal axis. This can occur 2 to 7 days after the injection.

Viscosupplementation

Properties of hyaluronic acid

Hyaluronic acid is a polysaccharide chain made of repeating disaccharide units of N-acetylglucosamine and glucuronic acid. Type B synoviocytes, in the synovium, synthesize hyaluronic acid and secrete it into the joint space. Hyaluronic acid is made of approximately 12,500 disaccharide units resulting in a molecular weight of 5×10^6 daltons. The human knee contains 2 mL of synovial fluid, with a concentration of hyaluronic acid of 2.5 to 4.0 mg/mL.

In osteoarthritis, the concentration and molecular weight of hyaluronic acid is reduced. There is a decreased interaction between the hyaluronic acid molecules, which results in lowering the viscosity and elastic properties of the synovial fluid. The lower viscosity creates increased stress forces, which can permanently damage the delicate articular cartilage. The lower viscosity creates an environment that reduces the barrier and filter effects of the synovial fluid. This reduces the nutrient availability and waste removal functions that are vital for the survival of articular cartilage.

Hyaluronic acid has both viscous and elastic properties. At high shear forces, hyaluronic acid exhibits increased elastic properties and reduced viscosity. The opposite is true with low shear forces. Therefore, hyaluronic acid acts as a shock absorber during fast movements, and a lubricant during slow movement. Hyaluronic acid also has several antiinflammatory effects by inhibiting phagocytosis and adherence of leukoctyes. It reduces the levels of inflammatory mediators such as prostaglandin and cyclic adenosine monophosphate. Hyaluronic acid also reduces the release of arachidonic acid from synovial fibroblasts. Arachidonic acid is usually taken up by synovial leukocytes and converted into inflammatory mediators. The reduction of the release of arachidonic acid by hyaluronic acid is dependent on the dose and molecular weight.

The intraarticular injection of hyaluronic acid may affect the synthesis of hyaluronic acid by synovial fibroblasts. Osteoarthritic joints produce a lower level of hyaluronic acid compared with normal joints. Smith et al studied the effect of different hyaluronic acid products on their ability to stimulate synovial fibroblasts [9]. The concentration and the molecular weight of hyaluronic acid were shown to be essential for the hyaluronic acid production. A molecular weight of 5×10^5 daltons was most effective, but at a high concentration it can have an inhibitory effect on synovial fibroblasts.

Ghosh et al showed the direct analgesic effect of hyaluronic acid in a rat model [10]. Intraarticular hyaluronic acid was found to be equivalent to indomethacin in reducing pain. The authors proposed that hyaluronic acid modulates pain by directly inhibiting nociceptors or indirectly binding substance P, which is involved in pain signals.

The chondroprotective effects of hyaluronic acid has not been clinically proven. There have been several animal studies supporting the chondroprotective effect of hyaluronic acid. In a canine model, osteoarthritis was induced by transection of the anterior cruciate ligament; there was an increase in matrix production that included hyaluronic acid [11]. In a sheep model, osteoarthritis was induced by medial and lateral meniscectomies, five weekly injections of hyaluronic acid inproved gait [12]. The injections did not prevent the progression of osteophyte formation and cartilage degeneration.

Viscosupplements

The use of hyaluronic acid for viscosupplementation began in the late 1960s by Biotrics, Inc. (Arlington, Massachusetts). The source material was taken from human umbilical cord and rooster combs. The hyaluronic acid could be purified, and was initially injected into race horses after traumatic injuries. In recent years, developers have targeted several properties that are important for the human application of hyaluronic acid. These properties are a lack of immunogenicity, capability of allowing passive diffusion within the synovial fluid, native rheologic properties, and a prolonged half-life within the synovium [1].

The hyaluronic acid products that are available in the United States are Synvisc (Biomatrix, Ridgeford, New Jersey), Hyalgan (Sanofi, New York, New York), and Supartz (Seika-gaku, Falmouth, Massachusetts). They are approved for use in patients with osteoarthritis of the knee. These products are derived from rooster combs; then the hyaluronic acid is purified and the noninflammatory hyaluronan product is isolated. The Food and Drug Administrations classifies viscosupplements as medical devices; therefore, the difficult regulations of a drug are not applied to these products. Two other viscosupplements are available in Canada, which are called Orthovisc (Anika Therapeutics, Woburn, Massachusetts) and Neovisc (Stellar International London, Ontario, Canada).

The molecular weight of human hyaluronic acid is approximately 5×10^6 daltons. It has been proposed that there is an improved mechanism of action with a higher molecular weight of the hyaluronic acid. The theory is that the higher molecular weight will improve the viscoelastic properties and residence time within the joint space. The hyaluronic acid molecules can be crosslinked to increase their molecular weight. Synvisc is the only crosslinked viscosupplement that is available in the United States.

Clinical safety

Hyaluronic acid has approximately a 1% incidence of side effects per injection. The most common side effects are local reactions of the knee such as swelling, pain, and increased warmth. This type of reaction typically lasts for 1 to 2 days. More recently, several reports of granulomatous inflammation of the knee after injections of hyaluronic acid [13,14]. Puttick et al observed clinically significant local inflammatory reactions in 11% of injections (27% of patients) [14]. Other studies have reported 2% to 4% incidence of local inflammatory reations [15]. Chen et al reported on six cases of granulomatous inflammation of the knee following hyaluronic acid injections [13]. All patients had pain, swelling, and warmth within 48 hours after the injection. The swelling gradually resolved in 1 to 2 weeks. This severe reaction is most likely due to the inability of the synovium to digest or degrade the foreign hyaluronic acid. The authors finally stated that this pathologic response to an intraarticular injection of hyaluronic acid should raise the clinical awareness of the potential complications of viscosupplementation.

Clinical results

There have been numerous studies evaluating the efficacy of hyaluronic acid for the treatment of osteoarthritis. Most of the studies have compared hyaluronic acid to placebo or corticosteroid injections, and the results have been variable. Dixon et al found that injections of hyaluronic acid over a 23-week period showed statistically significant improvement in knee pain at rest [16]. There was no improvement in pain with movement or activities of daily living. Dougados et al found that hyaluronic acid is significantly better than placebo for pain relief and improvement of the Lequesne functional index [17]. The group receiving the hyaluronic acid also had a significantly reduced need for treatment at 1 year.

In a large double-blind trial with Hyalgan, Altman et al found a significant benefit compared with placebo for the primary outcome in an efficacy analysis [18]. The efficacy analysis was performed on only the patients that completed the study. They also measured the Western Ontario and McMaster Universities Osteoarthritis Index (WOMAC) and found a significant improvement of pain and disability based on the WOMAC scores. Wobig et al performed a study on patients receiving hyaluronic acid and had their NSAID's discontinued for the project [19]. The authors found that hyaluronic acid was significantly more effective than placebo. In a 12-week study by Scale et al, the authors demonstrated a significant improvement in pain, activity, and patient/doctor global assessment [20]. They also found a significant improvement with a three-injection regimen compared with a two-injection regimen.

Jones et al reported on 63 patients that were prospectively randomized to receive hyaluronic acid or a corticosteroid injection for inflammatory knee arthritis [21]. The patients receiving hyaluronic acid reported less pain at 6 months than the steroid group. The study had 68.3% of the patients, from both groups, withdraw from the study due to worsening symptoms. A more recent study by Leopold et al, also compared hyaluronic acid to corticosteroid injections in a prospective, randomized trial [22]. The results showed no significant difference between the two treatment groups with respect to WOMAC, Knee society system, or visual analog scale results. The average follow-up was 6 months for this study, so long-term anaylsis was not performed.

Dahlberg et al performed the only study to date on the use of intraarticular hyaluronic acid on patients with early arthritis [23]. The study was a 52-week trial of hyaluronic acid in patients with normal knee radiographs. The patients had clinically significant knee pain and arthroscopically had evidence of early arthritis. There was no clinical benefit of injecting hyaluronic acid compared with placebo. This study did not support the use of hyaluronic acid in young patients, but supports further research on the use of viscosupplementation on patients with purely arthroscopic cartilage injuries.

An extensive meta-analysis of randomized controlled trials was performed by Wang et al on the effect of hyaluronic acid on osteoarthritis of the knee [24]. They found that single-blind and single-center design resulted in higher estimates in the efficacy of hyaluronic acid. They also found that when acetaminophen was introduced as an escape analgesic, there were lower estimates in the efficacy of hyaluronic acid. Last, they concluded that patients over the age of 60 and with advanced radiographic stage osteoarthritis (loss of joint space) were less likely to benefit from intraarticular hyaluronic acid injections. Therefore, the authors concluded that hyaluronic acid can significantly improve pain and functional outcomes with few adverse effects, but well-designed randomized controlled trials need to be continued.

Summary

There are many stages of osteoarthritis, in various locations, and in different patient populations. Corticosteroids have been used for many years in the treatment of osteoarthritis. They are relatively inexpensive and safe, but do not have clear, long-term benefits, and can damage collagen structures surrounding joints. Orthopedic surgeons need to continue to use corticosteroids cautiously and conservatively. As older patients increase their activity and demand on their joints, there needs to be further research into the value and efficacy of hyaluronic acid for osteoarthritis of the knee. Future projects should also incorporate the subset of patients with arthroscopic evidence of cartilage injury without radiographic changes. These patients have a larger amount of native articular cartilage in their joints compared with late stage osteoarthritis, which may enhance the effects of intraarticular hyaluronic acid. The research also needs to expand the use of hyaluronic acid to other joints effected by osteoarthritis such as the hip, shoulder, elbow, and ankle. In conclusion, hyaluronic acid injections should be limited until more convincing data on their efficacy are available from well-designed clinical trials.

References

[1] Watterson JR, Esdaile JM. Viscosupplementation: therapeutic mechanisms and clinical potential in osteoarthritis of the knee. J Am Acad Orthop Surg 2000;8(5):277–84.

[2] Hollander JL, Brown EM, Jessar RA, Brown CY. Comparative effects of and use of hydrocortisone as a local antiarthritic agent. JAMA 1951;147:1629–35.

[3] Rozental TD, Sculco TP. Intra-articular corticosteroids: an updated overview. Am J Orthop 2000;29:18–23.

[4] Rydell N, Balazs EA. Effect of intra-articular injection of hyaluronic acid on the clinical symptoms of osteoarthritis and on granulation tissue formation. Clin Orthop 1971;80:25–32.

[5] Youssef PP, Conmack J, Evill CA, et al. Neutrophil trafficking into inflamed joints in patients with rheumatoid arthritis, and the effects of methylprednisolone. Arthritis Rheum 1996;39(2): 216–25.

[6] Doherty M. Intra-articular corticosteroids are effective in osteoarthritis but there are no clinical predictors of response. Ann Rheum Dis 1996;55(11):829–32.

[7] Freidman DM, Moore MF. The efficacy of intraarticular steroids in osteoarthritis: a double blind study. J Rheumatol 1980;7:850–6.

[8] Stahl S, Kaufman T. The efficacy of an injection of steroids for medial epicondylitis. A prospective study of sixty elbows. J Bone Joint Surg 1997;79(11):1648–52.

[9] Smith MM, Ghosh P. The synthesis of hyaluronic acid by human synovial fibroblasts is influenced by the nature of the hyaluronate in the extracellular environment. Rheumatol Int 1987;7:113–22.

[10] Ghosh P. The role of hyaluronic acid (hyaluronan) in health and disease: interactions with cells, cartilage, and components of synovial fluid. Clin Exp Rheumatol 1994;12:75–82.

[11] Smith GN, Myers SL, Brandt KD, Mickler EA. Effect of intraarticular hyaluronan injection in experimental canine osteoarthritis. Arthritis Rheum 1998;41:976–85.

[12] Ghosh P, Read R, Armstrong S, Wilson D, Marshall R, McNair P. The effects of intra-articular administration of hyaluronan in a model of early osteoarthritis in sheep: I Gait analysis and radiological and morphological studies. Semin Arthritis Rheum 1993;22(6):18–30.

[13] Chen AL, Desai P, Adler EM, DiCesare PE. Granulomatous inflammation after hylan G-F 20 viscosupplementation of the knee: a report of six cases. J Bone Joint Surg 2002; 84-A(7):1142–7.

[14] Puttick MPE, Wade JP, Chalmers A, Connell DG, Rangno KK. Acute local reactions after intraarticular hylan for osteoarthritis of the knee. J Rheumatol 1995;22:1311–4.

[15] Peyron JG. Intraarticular hyaluronan injections in the treatment of osteoarthritis: state of the art review. J Rheumatol 1993;20(39):10–5.

[16] Dixon AS, Jacoby RK, Berry H, Hamilton EBD. Clinical trial of intra-articular injection of sodium hyaluronate in patients with osteoarthritis of the knee. Curr Med Res Opin 1988;11: 205–13.

[17] Dougados M, Nguyen M, Listrat V, Amor B. High molecular weight sodium hyaluronate (hyalectin) in osteoarthritis of the knee: A 1 year placebo-controlled tiral. Osteoarthritis Cartilage 1993;1:97–103.

[18] Altman RD, Moskowitz R. Hyalgan study group: intraarticular sodium hyaluronate (Hyalgan) in the treatment of patients with osteoarthritis of the knee: a randomized clinical trial. J Rheumatol 1998;25:2203–12.

[19] Wobig M, Dickut A, Maier R, Vetter G. Viscosupplementation with hyalan G-F 20: a 26-week controlled trial of efficacy and safety in the osteoarthritic knee. Clin Ther 1998;20:410–23.

[20] Scale D, Wobig M, Wolpert W. Viscosupplementation of osteoarthritic knees with hylan: a treatment schedule study. Curr Ther Res 1994;55:220–32.

[21] Jones AC, Pattrick M, Doherty S, Doherty M. Intra-articular hyaluronic acid compared to intra-articular triamcinolone hexacetonide in inflammatory knee osteoarthritis. Osteoarthritis Cartilage 1995;3:269–73.

[22] Leopold SS, Redd BB, Warme WJ, Wehrle PA, Pettis PD, Shott S. Corticosteroid compared with hyaluronic acid injections for the treatment of osteoarthritis of the knee: a prospective, randomized trial. J Bone Joint Surg 2003;85-A(7):1197–203.

[23] Dahlberg L, Lohmander LS, Ryd L. Intraarticular injections of hyaluronan in patients with cartilage abnormalities and knee pain: a one-year double-blind, placebo-controlled study. Arthritis Rheum 1994;37:521–8.

[24] Wang CT, Lin J, Chang CJ, Lin YT, Hou SH. Therapeutic effects of hyaluronic acid on osteoarthritis of the knee: a meta-analysis of randomized controlled trials. J Bone Joint Surg 2004;86-A(3):538–45.

[25] Lee S, Park D, Chmell SJ. Viscosupplementation with hylan G-F 20 (Synvisc): pain and mobility observations from 74 consecutive patients. J Knee Surg 2004;17(2):73–7.

ELSEVIER
SAUNDERS

Clin Sports Med 24 (2005) 93–99

CLINICS
IN SPORTS
MEDICINE

Orthotic and Brace Use in the Athlete with Degenerative Joint Disease with Angular Deformity

Andrew L. Pruitt, ATC, PA, EdD

Boulder Center for Sports Medicine, 311 Mapleton Avenue, Boulder, CO 80304, USA

The cost to society from lower extremity arthritis is enormous. The psychologic cost to the individual sufferer can be catastrophic. The numbers are huge; 17 to 20 million Americans are affected [1]. One source says 90% of adults over the age of 40 suffer at least occasionally from arthritic symptoms, so trying to fight the advancement of osteoarthritis is an important battle.

The word "orthotic" has become synonymous with prescription and nonprescription shoe inserts used to treat a number of common foot, knee, and back problems. The word "orthotic" in the truest medical sense means to straighten or correct function. So any device or technique used to treat the pain and dysfunction of angular deformity is an orthotic. The angular deformity does not have to be obvious to the naked eye. The word "orthotic" would include corrective shoes, knee braces, therapeutic taping, shoe insert, patellar tracking sleeves, hip spica, braces, etc.

The scope of this article is meant to cover the use of shoe inserts and knee braces to restore function for those with angularly deformed degenerative joint disease (DJD) of the ankle and knee. (In a perfect world when a body stands erect on both feet equally, the line of weight-bearing falls from the center of the femoral head, through the center of the knee, to the center of the ankle. In individuals where the lower extremity posture deviates from the perfect norm, gravitational forces are not dissipated correctly, and a breakdown in the articular cartilage can occur. This deviation from the perfect norm may be a result of congenital factors, trauma, or articular cartilage wear. The knee best illustrates the contribution of poor alignment to osteoarthritis [2–5].) The forces transmitted

E-mail address: andrew@hotmail.com

through the knee are thought to vary from three times body weight to as high as 10× body weight, depending on the velocity and mass involved with each heel strike; therefore, it is easily seen why it is important to maintain or restore proper lower extremity alignment [6–8]. Achieving better alignment may add years of active lifestyle and prevent or postpone the need for operative intervention. However, sometimes the surgeon, and only the surgeon, can recreate proper alignment.

In the author's 30 years as an athletic trainer and physician assistant, he has used and seen the benefits of orthotics to support or achieve lower extremity alignment improvement. Arthritis is not necessarily a disease of relentless progression if balance is achieved. A simple shoe insert that corrects malalignment can affect the ankle, knee, hip, and low back.

Foot orthoses

There is a real art to the creation of functional foot orthoses. It requires a thorough understanding of the lower extremity biomechanics. We must always remind ourselves that there is no free lunch; if we take pressure off of one structure, we will put it on another. Gravity cannot be eliminated, but it can be fooled.

For midfoot or ankle DJD, an orthotic can be very useful. With midfoot arthritis, just a simple arch support can be extremely helpful. With ankle arthritis, a canted orthotic can be employed if there is an area of talus that can be loaded or unloaded to achieve better alignment or pain relief. Anterior talar lesions often

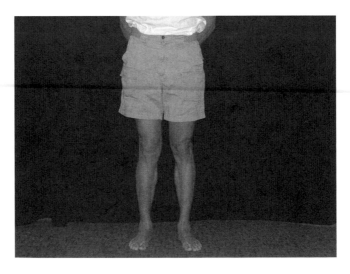

Fig. 1. Patient with gross valgus deformity.

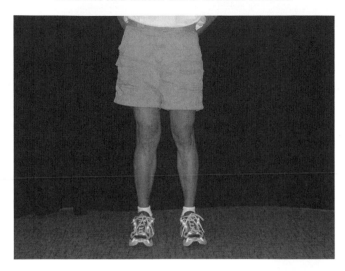

Fig. 2. Patient with aggressive varus posted orthotic.

respond well to a simple heel lift to open up the anterior joints. Although similar is true with a posterior lesion (including entrapment of the os trigonum), it can benefit from the reverse heel such as an earth shoe. The clever orthotist can combine fore, mid, and rearfoot correction to achieve good midstance balance and adjustment.

Foot orthotics can be used to treat angular deformity at the knee as well. They can be very effective in treatment of patellofemoral pain that is based on malalignment (Figs. 1–3).

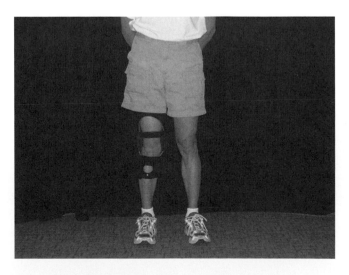

Fig. 3. Patient with orthotic plus varus unloader brace.

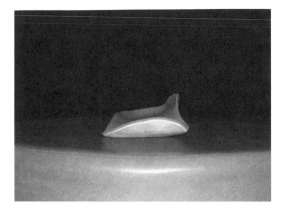

Fig. 4. Anterior–posterior view of orthotic.

It is common in the author's practice to have patients who use just in-shoe orthotics for activities of daily living and then combine with a knee brace for high-level activities.

Several studies have shown that even simple heel or sole wedges can be effective in reducing painful knee and ankle symptoms. Keating et al [2] reported 50% of subjects had good to excellent results with 5° lateral heel wedges in the treatment of moderate medial joint DJD. Yashuda and Sasaki [9] reported in 1985 that wedged insoles made no difference in the mechanical alignment of the knee, but by canting the calcaneus to valgus at the subtalar joint, load at the medial knee joint could be reduced, therefore, decreasing symptoms of DJD in that design of knee.

The prescribing practitioner must communicate their prescriptive wishes to the fabricator of the orthotic, but the patient is going to be the best source of information as to its usefulness and tolerance potential. The author has had patients who have more than one pair of orthotics with different corrections,

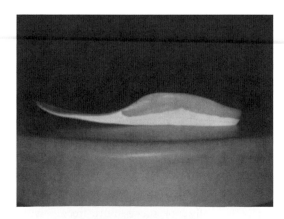

Fig. 5. Medial view of orthotic.

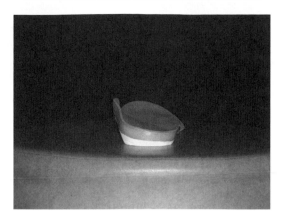

Fig. 6. Posterior–anterior view of orthotic.

and they use them all, as they find many times the loaded structures like to change or shift the load periodically. They might trade at noon or every other day to achieve comfort and tolerance. There are many different types of materials being used to fabricate orthotics, ranging from carbon fiber (rigid) to layers of varying density foams (soft or flexible), and all combinations in between. There is no right answer to the question of best material, but the author does have his favorites. He believes in semirigid orthotics. They must have enough structure to achieve the desired control at heel strike, midstance, and push-off phases. It is the author's belief that a one-piece rigid orthotic cannot do all three. Mindfully, he uses polyethylene as a basis for his orthotics. It has some torsional life to be able to move with the foot, but enough structure for control at the important midstance. Crepe or some other form of closed cell foam for rearfoot and forefoot postings works well. They do wear faster than rigid plastic, but perform better during the life of the orthotic (Figs. 4–6).

Mechanical knee orthoses (braces)

Osteoarthritis of the knee can be present in any of the three articular compartments of the knee and on one or both of the surfaces in those compartments. The most common site of initial degeneration is the medial compartment because the medial femoral condyle is typically longer than the lateral condyle; therefore, more forces both compressive and rotational are transferred in the medial compartment. Sixty percent to 80% of the transferred load crosses in the medial joint. This contributes to varus deformity. Varus deformity caused by lateral compartment degeneration is less often seen, and can be treated by braces/orthotics as well [10,11]. DJD seen equally in both medial and compartments is typically not successfully treated with bracing or foot orthoses. Patellofemoral DJD is not successfully treated with mechanical braces, although there are some tracking braces that some find useful if the DJD is limited to one facet of the patella or one side of the trochlear groove.

Ligament instability, even mild, can contribute to dynamic angular deformity and increase painful symptoms. Bracing can be a positive factor, if instability and angular deformity are combined due to the confinement components of bracing. An additional benefit of bracing is the improvement of proprioception in unstable knees.

Current technology is such as to try to reduce compression and shearing loads on the affected compartment. This load shift is achieved through a three-point force system. This three-point force system is applied to the knee through the medial/lateral plane. With medial compartment degeneration (varus deformity), a valgus force is applied and with lateral compartment degeneration (valgus deformity), a varus force is applied. These applied forces can shift the pressure from the degenerative compartment to the lesser worn compartment [3,4,12,13].

In cadaver and computer model studies, commercial braces have proven to effectively change the joint pressures and even affect joint space dramatically with excellent reproducibility. However, tolerance by real patients of these medial/lateral forces to the knee and on soft tissues is variable.

Horloch and Lomer reported in 1993 significant increases in function and decrease in pain with the use of what has become know as "unloader braces" [4]. Pallo et al reported a reduced external varus moment at the knee while walking, and this finding translated into a reduction of load in the degenerative compartment [5].

Summary

The use of heel wedges, angled shoe soles, in-shoe inserts (orthotics), and mechanical knee braces can be an effective treatment for degenerative angular deformities of the lower extremities. The improvement in lower extremity alignment may also have a positive effect on the hip and low back. However, orthotics and braces are not for everyone. Real patients may not tolerate the changes in lower extremity alignment or the counter pressures and forces placed on other tissues to unload degenerative tissues. Orthotics and braces should be considered early in treatment along with other noninvasive techniques.

References

[1] Brandt KD. Nonsurgical management of osteoarthritis with an emphasis on non-pharmacologic measures. Arch Fam Med 1995;4:1057–64.

[2] Keating EM, Farris PM, Ritter MA, Kane J. Use of lateral heel and sole wedges in the treatment of medial osteo arthritis of the knee. Ortho Rev 1993;22:921–41.

[3] Matsuno H, Kadowaki KM, Tsuji H. Generation II knee bracing for severe medial osteoarthritis of the knee. Arch Phys Med Rehabil 1997;78:745–9.

[4] Paulos LE. Case report: pain relief and functional improvement with use of the donjoy oadjuster knee brace. Vista (CA): DJ Orthopedics Biomechanics Lab.

[5] Pollo FE. Bracing and heel wedging for unicompartmental osteoarthritis of the knee. Am J Knee Surg 1998;11(1):47–50.

[6] Harrelson GL. Physiologic factors of rehabilitation. In: Andrews RA, Harrelson GL, editors. Physical rehabilitation of the injured athlete. Philadelphia: WB Saunders; 1991. p. 13–34.

[7] Nicholas JA, Hershman EB. The aging athlete and osteoarthritis of the knee. The lower extremity & spine in sports medicine. Vol. 1. St. Louis: Mosby; 1986. p. 790–800.

[8] Simon SR. Form and function of articular cartilage. In: Orthopaedic basic science. Rosemont (IL): American Academy of Orthopaedic Surgeons; 1994. p. 17–41.

[9] Yasuda K, Sasaki T. The mechanics of treatment of the osteoarthritic knee with a wedged insole. Clin Orthop 1987;215:162–72.

[10] Basic principles of knee rehabilitation; the chemical basis of tissue repair. In: Hunter LY, Funk Jr JF, editors. Rehabilitation of the injured knee. St. Louis: Mosby; 1995. p. 175–81.

[11] Snider RK. Essentials of musculoskeletal care: injections and corticosteroids. In: American Academy of Pediatrics. Section 1. General Orthopaedics. Rosemont (IL): American Academy of Orthopaedic Surgeons; 2001. p. 37–9.

[12] Barnes CL, Cawley PW, Hederman B. Effect of CounterForce brace on symptomatic relief in a group of patients with symptomatic unicompartmental osteoarthritis: a prospective 2-year investigation. Am J Orthoped 2000;31(7):396–401.

[13] Hewitt TE, Noyes FR, Barer-Westin SD, Heckman TP. Decrease in knee joint pain and increase in function in patients with medial compartment arthrosis: a prospective analysis of valgus bracing. Orthopedics 1998;21(2):131–8.

CLINICS
IN SPORTS
MEDICINE

Clin Sports Med 24 (2005) 101–131

Rehabilitation of the Osteoarthritic Patient: Focus on the Knee

Robert T. Bashaw, PT, SCS, OCS, ATC, CSCS[a],
Edwin M. Tingstad, MD[b],*

[a]Department of Intercollegiate Athletics, Washington State University, 825 SE Bishop Boulevard,
Suite 120, Pullman, WA 99163, USA
[b]Department of Orthopaedics and Sports Medicine, University of Washington,
1959 N.E. Pacific Street, Seattle, WA 98195, USA

Osteoarthritis (OA) is steadily becoming the most common cause of disability for the middle aged and has become the most common cause of disability for those over the age of 65 [1–8]. The desire to remain physically active for an aging population has led to an increasing need to prevent and rehabilitate the patient with degenerative joint disease. This article reviews some of the factors involved in the care and rehabilitation of the osteoarthritic patient, with emphasis on the knee.

The goal of rehabilitation in the patient who has OA is to improve function, minimize discomfort, and limit further injury. This tends to be a multifactorial process involving patient education, obtaining acceptable pain control, optimizing range of motion of the entire kinetic chain, functional strengthening of involved extremity, aerobic exercise, and use of assistive devices and orthoses [9]. This article will review the knee as an example of the process that seeks to protect, then unload the affected joint through a rehabilitative process. We emphasize to our patients that this process takes on more of the character of a marathon rather than a sprint.

Reviewing the pathophysiology of OA with the patient and the undulating and at times unpredicatable course that is commonly seen is an important part of patient education. Explaining the rationale for specific treatments helps to reinforce the need for a sustained program with goals. Encouraging the patient to

---

* Corresponding author.
E-mail address: tingstad@u.washington.edu (E.M. Tingstad).

take an active role in their rehabilitation process enhances compliance and shows promise in reducing pain and health care costs while improving quality of life [10]. Due to the fact that OA is often asymptomatic in its initial stages and later becomes symptomatic as the disease process progresses means that many are not seen until they have significant wear. Signs and symptoms of end-stage OA include severe pain, loss of motion and movement of the involved joint and limb, deformity, joint effusion, abnormal gait mechanics, and activity of daily living lifestyle changes and compensations. A review of the signs, symptoms and natural history of OA with the patient is helpful as it gives them a better understanding of what to expect and the rationale for their therapy. Common in all OA conditions is an overload of a focal area of articular cartilage, which leads to failure of the load-bearing capacity of the cartilage and subchondral bone [11]. The analagy of "building a better shock absorber" is one that most patients seem to enjoy and understand.

Pain control is an important early goal. The use of medications, cryotherapy, heat, and orthoses all assist in minimizing discomfort. Furthermore, the use of intra-articular injections, acetaminophen, anti-inflammatories, and glucosamine all have been shown to reduce pain [12]. Coordination of these with activity and exercise allows judicious use and more productive therapy. Cryotherapy has been shown by many authors to reduce pain, intra-articular temperature, and inflammatory mediator release [13]. Patient education also contributes in this area as reviewing the fact that exercise increases circulating endorphins allows patients to understand that exercise can reduce the discomfort rather than increase pain by using the patients own protective capacity [14].

Ongoing patient education and analgesia allow for the initiation of a therapeutic program as the next step in the rehabilitation process. To decrease the risk of further joint injury and degeneration to the knee, several interventions should be implemented. First, sporting or recreational activities and exercise programs should be low impact and not include significant torsional loading to the knee. Examples include recreational swimming, stationary cycling, low-impact aerobics, golf, or walking [2,3,15,16]. It has also been suggested that the activities be alternated in a manner that decreases repetition of the same movement patterns and joint loads [17]. The use of an orthosis (eg, a cane) can reduce the muscle forces needed for ambulation [11], though many patients prefer not to use this assistive device. Secondly, exercises should be implemented to improve muscle strength, stability, and endurance to the trunk and lower extremities to help the muscle's own ability to absorb impact and loads to the involved joint [18–33]. Lastly, general conditioning should be performed to help maintain desired weight and decrease the risk of joint injury due to fatigue [34,35].

Weight reduction through proper diet and aerobic exercise for the overweight patient is recommended to decrease joint loads to the osteoarthritic knee. However, no randomized control trial has shown that weight loss alone treats OA in a sustained fashion. Forces of 3 to 8 times body weight act on the knee with weight bearing activites [11]. Huang and colleagues [35] looked at the effects of weight reduction on the rehabilitation of patients with knee OA and obesity. They found that there was pain reduction, weight reduction, and improved ambulation speed in patients who were participating in a weight loss program. It is generally accepted that weight loss can occur with sustained aerobic activities lasting more that 20 minutes at a target heart rate in the range of 50% to 85% of maximal heart rate. Aerobic exercise should be performed at least three times per week [36]. Exercises should be of low-level joint loading such as walking, stationary cycling, low-impact aerobics, or swimming. Low impact is emphasized as those with joint disease have 30% less shock-absorbing capacity when compared with healthy controls [37]. Adequate muscular strength and stability during stance phase in gait and with other activities of daily living offers the patient with OA the means to attenuate forces going through the knee caused by momentum, ground reactive forces, and gravity. Thus, it is important that patients be taught functional strengthening and balance exercises to allow the greater symptom-fee activity.

The goal of the therapeutic program is to offset detrimental and inefficient biomechanical issues about the knee and entire kinetic chain. Thus, as appropriate diagnosis and an understanding of the causative factors allow the design of a therapeutic exercise program that can reduce the abnormal compressive loads to the joint.

Human movement is created and influenced by momentum, ground reaction forces, and gravity [38]. All joints in the body move through varying degrees of movement in all three planes of motion (sagittal, frontal, transverse) at once. The muscles functionally control the joint movements by decelerating motion by eccentrically elongating, and stabilizing the joints at the loaded transitional phase through isometric contraction and accelerating movements by shortening or concentric contraction to allow the body to perform those movements necessary to allow for normal locomotor motion [39]. Angular bone deformities or muscular imbalances can lead to focal joint overload over time and predispose the joint to osteoarthritic changes [39].

Common angular deformities about the knee include varus and valgus deformities and flexion contractures. Varus deformities causes overload to the medial knee compartment. Biomechanicaly, the knee joint is relatively extended in the sagittal plane, adducted in the frontal plane, and externally rotated in the transverse plane. Possible causes of knee varus deformity include uncompensated rear foot varus or uncompensated forefoot varus in which the foot is rigid and high arched or from a retroverted hip or tight hip external rotators. Sometimes, anatomically the tibia-femoral joint angle can produce a varus moment from past subchondral fractures that did not properly heal or other changes from joint incongruities or instabilities leading to compensations or meniscal derangements.

Conversely, valgus deformities cause overload to the lateral knee compartment. Biomechanically the knee assumes a position of flexion in the sagittal plane, abduction in the frontal plane and internal rotation in the transverse plane. Causative factors could include fully compensated forefoot varus deformity in the foot or increased foot pronation, anteverted hip or weakness of the hip external rotators or hip abductors, just to name a few.

Knee flexion contractures cause increased compressive forces to both the tibiofemoral and patellofemoral joints [24]. Maintenance of a static load promotes movement of fluid from articular cartilage into the joint space, reducing cartilaginous viscoelasticity [9,40]. Weight bearing on a knee flexion contracture can create pannus infiltration, erosion, and osteophyte formation on focal points on the medial and lateral femoral condyles corresponding to the areas normally in contact with the anterior horns of the menisci when the knee is in its extended position [41]. These changes support the work by Salter and McNeil [42] that degenerative changes can develop when articular cartilage is no longer in contact with an opposing surface.

Improved range of motion has been shown to improve discomfort and result in an increase in function [9,43,44]. Many authors have studied the differences in gait between normal patients and patients who have knee OA [45–47]. Their conclusions demonstrate that patients who have OA have decreased walking speed, shorter stride length, reduced peak vertical ground reaction forces, and longer stance phase compared with the control groups. These same patients had a

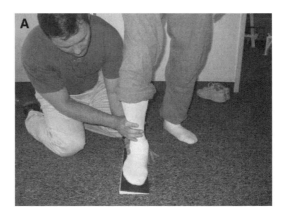

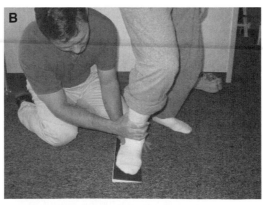

Fig. 1. Standing semi–weight bearing on lateral foot wedge subtalar and talocrural functional manual joint mobilizations. (*A*) Start position. (*B*) End position.

reduction in power in the ankle plantarflexors, and the quadriceps at terminal stance and greater power generated at the hip, knee, and ankle. They summarized that the lack of ankle plantarflexor power was due to disrupted transfer of energy through the knee and that patients with OA avoid using their quadriceps to stabilize their unstable knees, probably in an attempt to reduce articular loads to the joint. The increase in hip power was due to increased hip extension caused by abnormal knee kinematics. Patients with unilateral OA exhibit significantly reduced range of motion at lower limb joints bilaterally [48,49]. Thus, focusing on the entire kinetic chain becomes the key to protecting the arthritic joint (Figs. 1–4).

Practically, this requires a program that emphasizes a three-times-a-day program of stretching for seven sets of 15 to 20 seconds that includes the hips, knees, foot, and ankle. The exercises can be taught in a few visits, with the therapist and patient working together.

Strengthening becomes the next goal; this should be incorporated with the range of motion program. Range of motion is a prerequisite for functional

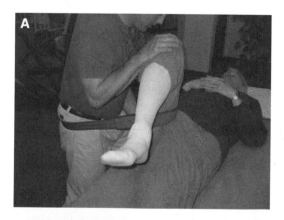

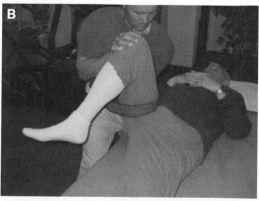

Fig. 2. Manual hip mobilization to help gain hip internal rotation using the Mulligan Concept. (A) Start position. (B) End position.

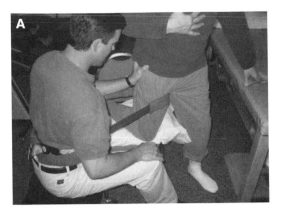

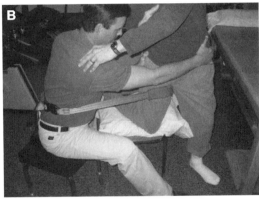

Fig. 3. Manual hip mobilization to help gain hip internal rotation using the Mulligan Concept. (*A*) Start position. (*B*) End position.

strengthening. Many studies have been performed to look at quadriceps weakness in patients who have OA [50–57]. Patients who have asymptomatic early radiographic arthritis show reduced quadriceps strength of 15% even when controlling for lean muscle mass in matched comparisons. These studies have shown that quadriceps weakness and peak torque values were significantly less in the OA groups tested. The degree of weakness may correlate with severity of the discomfort [56,58–60]. The weakness in this particular muscle group has been postulated to be either as a result of disease atrophy secondary to pain from the knee, or possibly due to primary dysfunction leading to functional weakness. This can place the knee at risk for pain, disability, and progression of joint damage if left untreated. Sensorimotor and knee joint proprioception has been looked at between control groups and groups with unilateral OA [61,62]. There was a reduction in quadriceps motorneuron excitability which not only contributed to decreases in quadriceps activation and strength, but also diminished proprioceptive activity and joint position sense. This led to a decline

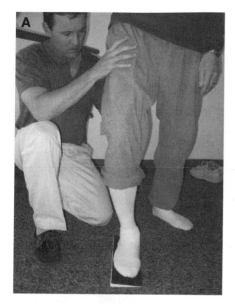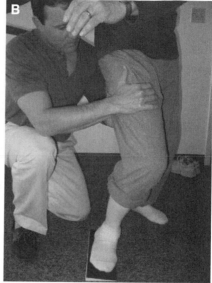

Fig. 4. Standing semi–weight bearing on a lateral foot wedge manual hip external rotation functional joint mobilizations. (*A*) Start position. (*B*) End position.

in the OA patient's postural stability and overall functional performance (Figs. 5–8).

Once again, in practical purposes, restoring range of motion with minimal discomfort followed by a strengthening program that incorporates the entire kinetic chain can be markedly helpful in restoring a patient's function. Based on the literature, focusing on quadriceps and hamstring strengthening is recommended. Initial isometric contractions may also help minimize early pain and give confidence. Straight leg raises, wall sits, isometric leg press are reasonable examples. Transition toward isotonic exercises are then begun such as squats, wall slides, leg press as long as isometrics are well tolerated. Aquatic therapy is incorporated as soon as possible, because it allows a resistive environment that may unload up to 50% to 60% of body weight [9].

Training programs that have focused on improving overall general fitness, balance, coordination, flexibility, lower extremity muscular strength, endurance, and overall function have been repeatedly shown to be effective [18–33]. All of the studies referenced above proved to be efficacious in symptom management and improved function in patients who had knee OA. Aerobic fitness programs specifically have been shown to reduce pain and morning stiffness, improve balance and walking speed, and enhance global function; this includes reducing depression and anxiety [63–66]. The benefits seem to last for an extended period.

In a study by Fisher and colleagues [18], 15 men who had diagnosed knee OA participated in a 4-month, three-times-per-week exercise program. The purpose of the study was to demonstrate the effect of a muscular rehabilitation program on

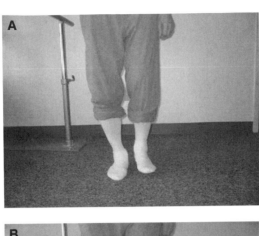

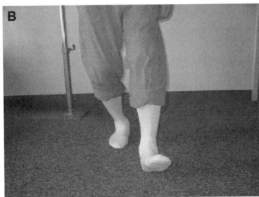

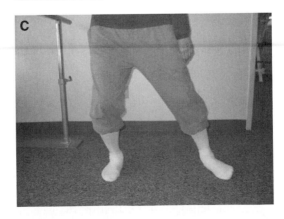

Fig. 5. One leg balance reach in all three planes of motion. (*A*) Start position. (*B*) Sagittal plane reach.
(*C*) Frontal plane reach. (*D*) Transverse plane reach.

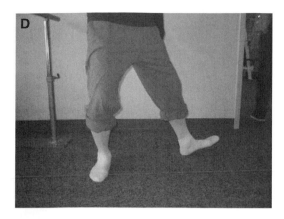

Fig. 5 (*continued*).

strength, endurance, speed, and function. They concluded that there was a significant increase in strength (35%), endurance (35%), and speed (50%). Furthermore, the improved muscular function led to a decrease in dependency (10%), difficulty of activities of daily living (30%), and pain (40%). The improvements were sustained for 8 months after completing the program.

The use of assistive devices and orthotics plays an ancillary role the rehabilitative process. Wedge insoles, functional braces, neoprene knee sleeves and assistive devices such as canes have all been shown to be beneficial. Kerrigan studied the use of a lateral wedge insole on patients who had knee varus torques and medial knee OA [67]. They concluded that 5- and 10-degree lateral wedge insoles significantly reduced knee varus torque during ambulation by 6% and 8%, respectively.

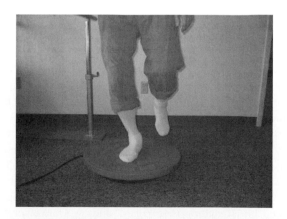

Fig. 6. One-leg proprioceptive balances.

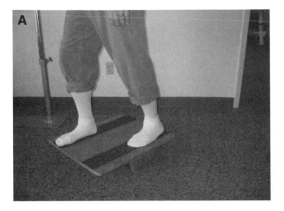

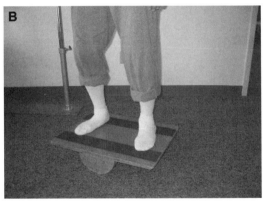

Fig. 7. Two-leg proprioceptive balances on balance board. (*A*) In the sagittal plane. (*B*) In the frontal plane.

In another study by Pollo and colleagues [68], they determined that valgus knee bracing was found to be beneficial in patients who had medial compartment OA. The bracing reduced the net varus moment about the knee by an average of 13% and the medial compartment load at the knee by an average of 11%. Thus, it appears that either lateral wedge insoles or dynamic knee bracing could be used to help decrease the stress to the medial joint compartment and help alleviate pain and improve the normal biomechanics of the knee joint (Figs. 9–13). Additionally, we have found that this faulty biomechanical knee position can be a result of a tight posterior and posterior–lateral hip complex, causing the femur to not flex, adduct, and internally rotate during the loading phase of gait. This causes the knee to remain relatively extended, abducted, and externally rotated, and could lead to medial joint overload over time. Treatment of this group includes hip mobilizations and hip stretching (see Figs. 2 and 3). Conversely, those patients who demonstrate lateral joint overload due to abnormal valgus knee deformity

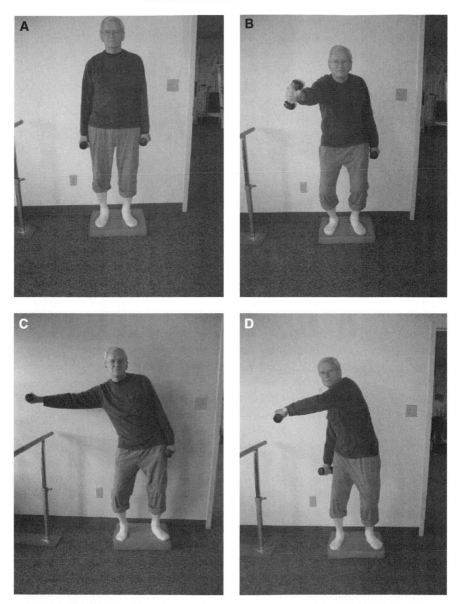

Fig. 8. Two-leg proprioceptive balances on Air-Ex balance pad with arm drivers. (*A*) Start position. (*B*) Arm drive in the sagittal plane. (*C*) Arm drive in the frontal plane. (*D*) Arm drive in the transverse plane.

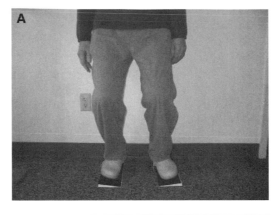

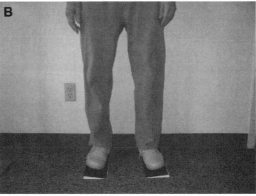

Fig. 9. Partial bilateral squats on lateral foot wedges. (*A*) Start position. (*B*) End position.

may benefit from a medial forefoot wedge if the cause of the knee deformity is thought to be from overpronation due to an uncompensated fore foot varus deformity. Proximally, these patients tend to have dormant or weak posterior and posterior lateral hips that create excessive femoral flexion, adduction, and internal rotation at initial contact. Valgus knee deformity patients should have an exercise program to improve the strength and endurance of the hip and core to better control the femur at the knee (Figs. 14–18). Focal overloading caused by weight bearing on a flexion-contracted knee can accelerate the degenerative process [11]. The aggressive physical therapy should include joint mobilizations if appropriate and passive- and active-assisted range of motion exercises. Long-leg knee immobilizer bracing could also be used to impart a prolonged knee extension stretch during the day or night. Restoring the knee to full extension enlarges the weight bearing contact of the femur on the tibia, thus decreasing the articular compressive forces (Figs. 19–25).

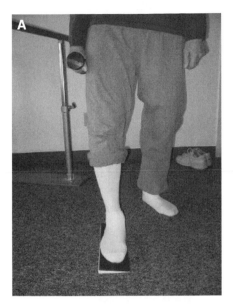 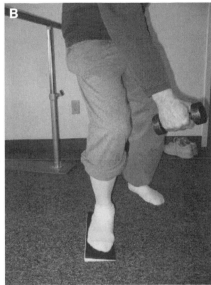

Fig. 10. Standing semi–weight bearing on lateral foot wedge with arm drive in transverse plane to help promote knee pronation. (*A*) Start position. (*B*) End position.

Shoe wear can also play an important role in the management of patients who have knee OA. Bone vibrations at 25 to 100 cycles per second at heel strike during gait have been measured [37,69]. Voloshin and Wosk [69] have shown that shock absorbing insoles resulted in a 42% reduction in the amplitude of shock waves during gait. They reported that 78% of the patients they followed had a disappearance in clinical symptoms of knee OA. It makes sense that those patients who work a lot while on their feet would benefit from shoes that are more forgiving and have better cushion than wearing shoes that are stiffer and have a hard sole. Kerrigan and colleagues [70] showed that women wearing high-heeled shoes had a 30% greater effect on peak knee flexor torque than walking barefoot. Thus, knee patients with OA should be advised to not wear high-heeled shoes.

Many authors [18–33] have studied the results of varied exercise programs assessing the reduction in pain and improvement of range of motion, strength, general fitness, and function. In a study performed by Gur and colleagues [23], they looked at concentric, isotonic strengthening versus combined concentric–eccentric isokinetic training on the effects of functional outcomes of patients with OA of the knee. Both groups showed a decrease in pain and increases in functional capacity of standing from a seated position, walking and ambulating up and down stairs. They also found that the concentric-eccentric group had a greater influence on functional capacity than the group who performed only concentric training. The program was 3 days per week for 8 weeks. In another study performed by Huang et al [22], they compared isokinetic versus isotonic

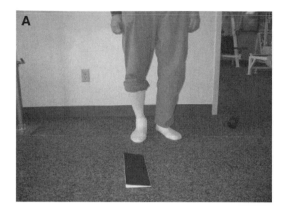

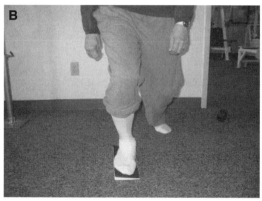

Fig. 11. (*A*) Start position for lunge on lateral foot wedge in sagittal plane. (*B*) End position for lunge on lateral foot wedge in sagittal plane.

and isometric strengthening. They found that each group had significant improvement in pain reduction, disability reduction, and walking speed after treatment and a 1-year follow-up. The isotonic exercise group had the greatest effect on reducing pain, and the isokinetic group had the greatest increase in walking speed and decrease of disability after treatment and follow-up. Lastly, Deyle and colleagues [29] performed manual physical therapy and exercise on 42 patients who had knee OA twice weekly for 4 weeks. The manual techniques were performed on the patient's affected knee, lumbar spine, hip, and ankle as required, and these techniques were combined with a standardized knee exercise program. They found a significant improvement in the distance walked in 6 minutes. These studies have consistently shown that a directed physical therapy program is an important and efficacious intervention in patients who have knee OA.

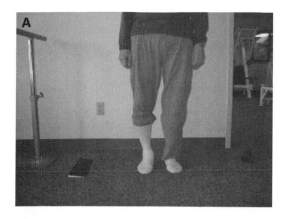

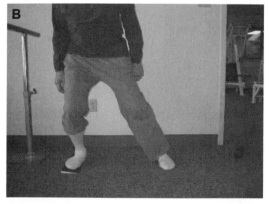

Fig. 12. (*A*) Start position for lunge on lateral foot wedge in frontal plane. (*B*) End position for lunge on lateral foot wedge in frontal plane.

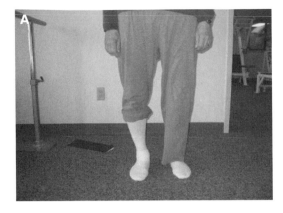

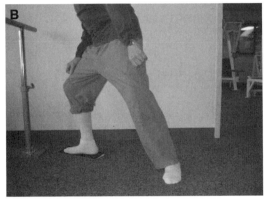

Fig. 13. (*A*) Start position for lunge on lateral foot wedge in transverse plane. (*B*) End position for lunge on lateral foot wedge in transverse plane.

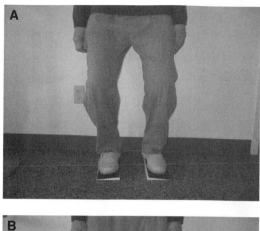

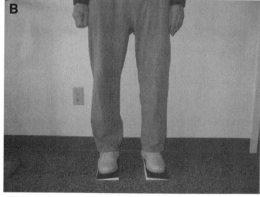

Fig. 14. Partial bilateral squats on medial foot wedges. (*A*) Start position. (*B*) End position.

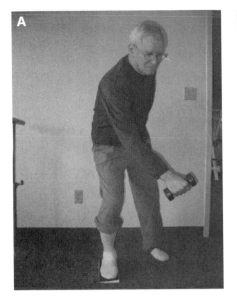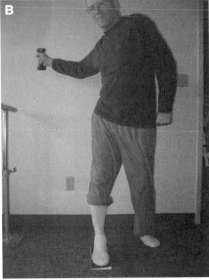

Fig. 15. Partial weight bearing on medial foot wedge using arm driver in transverse plane to help strengthen the hip and leg. (*A*) Start position. (*B*) End position.

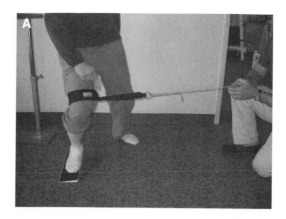

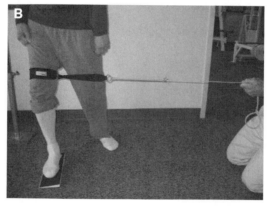

Fig. 16. Standing partial squats on a medial foot wedge in semi–weight bearing with tubing resistance to help strengthen the hip external rotators. (*A*) Start position. (*B*) End position.

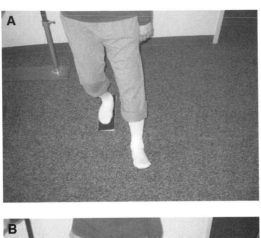

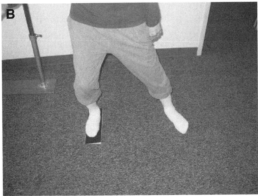

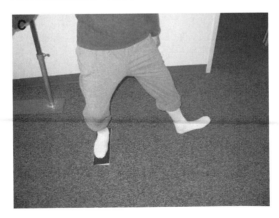

Fig. 17. One leg balance reach in all three planes of motion using a medial foot wedge. (*A*) Sagittal plane reach. (*B*) Frontal plane reach. (*C*) Transverse plane reach.

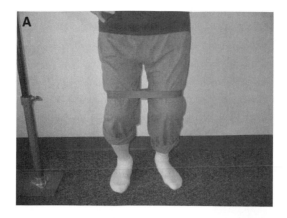

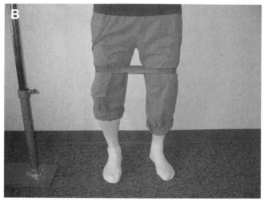

Fig. 18. Partial bilateral squats with band resistance for hip external rotation strengthening. (*A*) Start position. (*B*) End position.

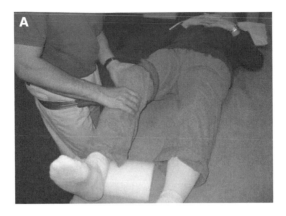

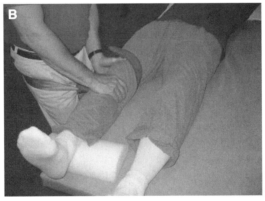

Fig. 19. Manual knee mobilization to help gain knee extension using the Mulligan Concept. (*A*) Start position. (*B*) End position.

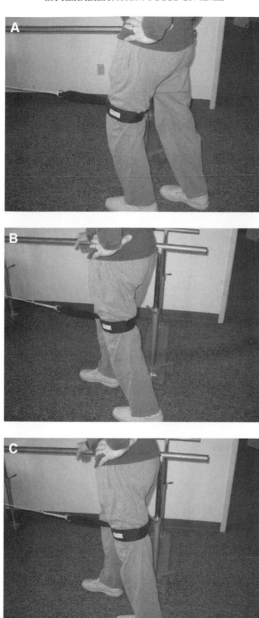

Fig. 20. Standing terminal knee extensions with walk-throughs using band resistance. (*A*) Start position. (*B*) Midstance position. (*C*) Terminal stance position.

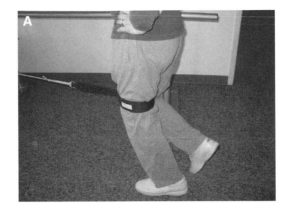

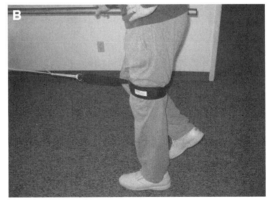

Fig. 21. Partial weight bearing terminal knee extensions. (*A*) Start position. (*B*) End position.

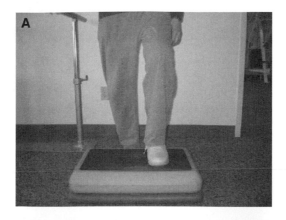

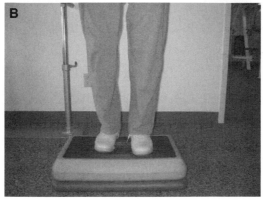

Fig. 22. (*A*) Start position for sagittal plane step up. (*B*) End position for sagittal plane step up.

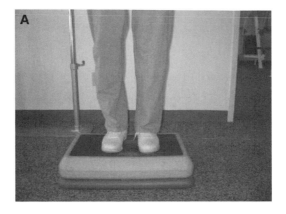

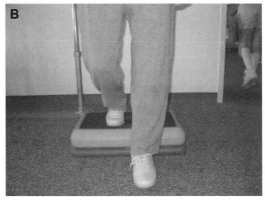

Fig. 23. (A) Start position for sagittal plane step down. (B) End position for sagittal plane step down.

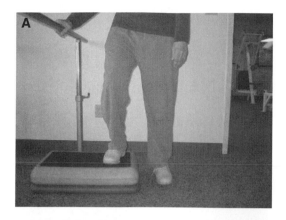

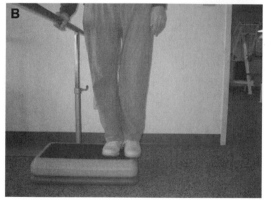

Fig. 24. (*A*) Start position for frontal plane step up. (*B*) End position for frontal plane step up.

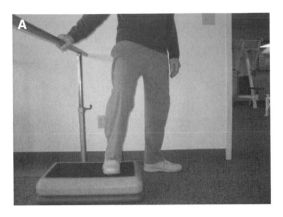

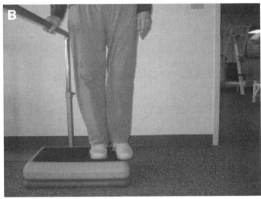

Fig. 25. (*A*) Start position for transverse plane step up. (*B*) End position for transverse plane step up.

Thus, a rehabilitation program directed at patient education, pain management, restoration of range of motion, and functional strengthening within the foundation of an aerobic fitness program give the patient and the treating clinician the tools necessary to help maintain an active and healthy lifestyle.

References

[1] Buckwalter JA. Articular cartilage injuries. Clin Orthop 2002;21–37.
[2] Buckwalter JA. Mechanical injuries of articular cartilage. In: Finerman G, editor. Biology and biomechanics of the traumatized synovial joint. Park Ridge (IL): American Academy of Orthopedic Surgeons; 1992. p. 83–96.
[3] Buckwalter JA, Lane NE. Athletics and osteoarthritis. Am J Sports Med 1997;25:873–81.
[4] Buckwalter JA, Mankin HJ. Articular cartilage I. Tissue design and chondrocyte-matrix interactions. J Bone Joint Surg 1997;79A:600–11.
[5] Buckwalter JA, Mankin HJ. Articular cartilage II. Degeneration and osteoarthritis, repair, regeneration, and transplantation. J Bone Joint Surg 1997;79A:612–32.

[6] Buckwalter JA, Martin J, Mankin HJ. Synovial joint degeneration and the syndrome of osteoarthritis. Instr Course Lect 2000;4:481–9.

[7] Cooper C, Snow S, McAlindon TE, Kellingray S, Stuart B, Coggon D, et al. Risk factors for the incidence and progression of radiographic knee osteoarthritis. Arthritis Rheum 2000; 43:995–1000.

[8] Buckwalter J, Martin J, Mankin H. Synovial joint degeneration and syndrome of osteoarthritis. Instr Course Lect 2000;49:481–9.

[9] Smith J. Physical therapy for early knee osteoarthritis. Mayo Clinic comprehensive review of upper and lower extremity. Mayo Press; 2001.

[10] Lorig K, Mazonson P, Holman H. Evidence suggesting that health education for self-management in patients with chronic arthritis has health benefits while reducing health care cost. Arthritis Rheum 1993;36:439–46.

[11] Nicholas J, Hershman E. Osteoarthrosis of the knee. In: Distefano VJ, editor. The lower extremity and spine in sports medicine. St. Louis (MO): C.V. Mosby; 1986. p. 881–90.

[12] Carlson S. Arthritis, orthopedic knowledge update. Rosemont (IL): American Academy of Orthopaedic Surgeon; 2002.

[13] Glenn RE, Spindler KP, Warren TA, Secic M. Cryotherapy decreased intraarticuluar temperature after ACL reconstruction. Clin Ortho 2004;421:268–72.

[14] Ekdahl C, Andersson S, Moritz U, Sversson B. Dynamic versus stasis training in patients with rheumatoid arthritis. Scand J Rheum 1990;19:17–26.

[15] Marsh JL, Buckwalter J, Gelberman R, Dirschl D, Olson S, Brown T, et al. Articular fractures: does an anatomic reduction really change the result? J Bone Joint Surg Am 2002;84-A:1259–71.

[16] Buckwalter JA. Osteoarthritis and articular cartilage use, disuse, and abuse: experimental studies. J Rheumatol Suppl 1995;43:13–5.

[17] Buckwalter JA. Sports, joint injury, and posttraumatic osteoarthritis. J Orthop Sports Phys Ther 2003;33:578–85.

[18] Fisher NM, Pendergast DR, Gresham GE, Calkins E. Muscle rehabilitation: its effect on muscular and functional performance of patients with knee osteoarthritis. Arch Phys Med Rehabil 1991;72:367–74.

[19] Baker K, McAlindon T. Exercise for knee osteoarthritis. Curr Opin Rheumatol 2000;12:456–63.

[20] Fransen M, McConnell S, Bell M. Exercise for osteoarthritis of the hip or knee. Cochrane Database System Review 2003;3:CD004286.

[21] Rogind H, Bibow-Nielsen B, Jensen B, Moller HC, Frimodt-Moller H, Bliddal H. The effects of a physical training program on patients with osteoarthritis of the knees. Arch Phys Med Rehabil 1998;79:1421–7.

[22] Huang MH, Lin YS, Yang RC, Lee CL. A comparison of various therapeutic exercises on the functional status of patients with knee osteoarthritis. Semin Arthritis Rheum 2003;32:398–406.

[23] Gur H, Cakin N, Akova B, Okay E, Kucukoglu S. Concentric versus combined concentric-eccentric isokinetic training: effects on functional capacity and symptoms in patient with osteoarthritis of the knee. Arch Phys Med Rehabil 2002;83:308–16.

[24] Eyigor S. A comparison of muscle training methods in patients with knee osteoarthritis. Clin Rheumatol 2004;23:109–15.

[25] Marks R. The effect of isometric quadriceps strength training in midrange for osteoarthritis of the knee. Arthritis Care Res 1993;6:52–6.

[26] Fisher NM, White SC, Yack HJ, Smolinski RJ, Pendergast DR. Muscle function and gait in patients with knee osteoarthritis before and after muscle rehabilitation. Disabil Rehabil 1997; 19:47–55.

[27] Rejeski WJ, Ettinger Jr WH, Martin K, Morgan T. Treating disability in knee osteoarthritis with exercise therapy: central role for self-efficacy and pain. Arthritis Care Res 1998;11:94–101.

[28] Borjesson M, Robertson E, Weidenhielm L, Mattsson E, Olsson E. Physiotherapy in knee osteoarthritis: effect on pain and walking. Physiotherapy Res Int 1996;1:89–97.

[29] Deyle GD, Henderson NE, Matekel RL, Ryder MG, Garber MB, Allison SC. Effectiveness of manual physical therapy and exercise in osteoarthritis of the knee. A randomized, controlled trial. Ann Intern Med 2000;132:173–81.

[30] Yurtkuran M, Kocagil T. TENS, electroacupuncture and ice massage: comparison of treatment for osteoarthritis of the knee. Am J Acupuncture 1999;27:133–40.

[31] Topp R, Woolley S, Hornyak 3rd J, Khuder S, Kahaleh B. The effect of dynamic versus isometric resistance training on pain and functioning among adults with osteoarthritis of the knee. Arch Phys Med Rehabil 2002;83:1187–95.

[32] Fitzgerald GK, Childs JD, Ridge TM, Irrgang JJ. Agility and perturbation training for a physically active individual with knee osteoarthritis. Phys Ther 2002;82:372–82.

[33] Wyatt FB, Milam S, Manske RC, Deere R. The effects of aquatic and traditional exercise programs on persons with knee osteoarthritis. J Strength Cond Res 2001;15:337–40.

[34] Felson DT, Zhang Y, Anthony JM, Naimark A, Anderson JJ. Weight loss reduces the risk for symptomatic knee osteoarthritis in women. The Framingham Study. Ann Intern Med 1992; 116:535–9.

[35] Huang MH, Chen CH, Chen TW, Weng MC, Wang WT, Wang YL. The effects of weight reduction on the rehabilitation of patients with knee osteoarthritis and obesity. Arthritis Care Res 2000;13:398–405.

[36] Williams MH. Weight maintenance and loss through proper nutrition and exercise. In: Rogers C, editor. Nutrition for fitness and sport. Dubuque (IA): William C. Brown Pub.; 1992.

[37] Voloshin A, Wosk J. Shock absorbing capacity of the human knee (in vivo properties). In: Proceedings of the Special Conference of the Canadian Society of Biomechanics on "Human Locomotion I." London, Ontario, Canada, 1980. p. 104.

[38] Gray G, Tiberio D. Chain reaction explosion seminar. Instr Course Lect 2001;1:11–27.

[39] Maquet P. Biomechanics of the knee with application to the pathogenesis and the surgical treatment of osteoarthritis. Berlin: Springer-Verlag; 1976.

[40] Norlein C, Lavangic P. Joint structure and function. Philadelphia: F.A. Davis; 1983.

[41] Waugh W, Newton G. Articular changes associated with flexion deformity in rheumatoid and osteoarthritic knees. J Bone and Joint Surg 1980;62B:180–3.

[42] Salter RB, McNeil R. Pathologic changes in articular cartilage secondary to persistent joint deformity. J Bone Joint Surg 1965;47B:185.

[43] Halar E, Bell K. Immobility. In: DeLisa J, Gans B, editors. Rehabilitation medicine: principles and practice. 3rd edition. Philadelphia: Lippincott-Raven; 1998. p. 1015–54.

[44] Minor M, Hinett J, Webel R, Anderson S, Kay D. Efficiency of physical condition exercise in patients with rheumatoid arthritis and osteoarthritis. Arthritis and Rheumatology 1989;32: 1396–405.

[45] Al-Zahrani KS, Bakheit AM. A study of the gait characteristics of patients with chronic osteoarthritis of the knee. Disabil Rehabil 2002;24:275–80.

[46] McGibbon CA, Krebs DE. Compensatory gait mechanics in patients with unilateral knee arthritis. J Rheumatol 2002;29:2410–9.

[47] Childs JD, Sparto PJ, Fitzgerald GK, Bizzini M, Irrgang JJ. Alterations in lower extremity movement and muscle activation patterns in individuals with knee osteoarthritis. Clin Biomechanics 2004;19:44–9.

[48] Messier S, et al. Osteoarthritis of the knee: effects on gait, strength, and flexibility. Arch Phys Med Rehabil 1993;73:29–36.

[49] Minor M. Exercise in the management of osteoarthritis of the knee and hip. Arthritis Care Res 1994;7:198–204.

[50] Slemenda C, Brandt KD, Heilman DK, Mazzuca S, Braunstein EM, Kat BP, et al. Quadriceps weakness and osteoarthritis of the knee. Ann Intern Med 1997;127:97–104.

[51] Fisher NM, Pendergast DR. Reduced muscle function in patients with osteoarthritis. Scand J Rehabil Med 1997;29:213–21.

[52] Wessel J. Isometric strength measurements of knee extensors in women with osteoarthritis of the knee. J Rheumatol 1996;23:328–31.

[53] Lewek MD, Rudolph KS, Snyder-Mackler L. Quadriceps femoris muscle weakness and activation failure in patients with symptomatic knee osteoarthritis. J Orthop Res 2004;22:110–5.

[54] Fransen M, Crosbie J, Edmonds J. Isometric muscle force measurement for clinicians treating patients with osteoarthritis of the knee. Arthritis Rheum 2003;49:29–35.

[55] Nakamura T, Suzuki K. Muscular changes in osteoarthritis of the hip and knee. Nippon Seikeigeka Gakkai Zasshi 1992;66:467–75.

[56] Slemenda C, Brandt K, Heilman D, Mazuca S, Braunstein E, Katz B, et al. Quadriceps weakness and osteoarthritis of the knee. Ann Int Med 1997;127:97–104.

[57] Hurley M, Newham D. The influence of autogenous muscle inhibition on quadricps rehabilitation of patients with early, unilateral osteoarthritic knees. Br J Rheumatol 1993;32: 127–31.

[58] Felson D, Amderson J, Naimark A, Walker A, Meenan R. Obesity and knee osteoarthritis. Ann Intern Med 1989;109:18–24.

[59] Tan J, Balci N, Sepici V, Gener F. Isokinetic and isometric strength in osteoarthritis of the knee: a comparative study with healthy women. Am J Phys Med Rehabil 1995;4:364–9.

[60] Nordesio L, et al. Isometric strength and endurance in patients with severe rheumatoid arthritis or osteoarthritis of the knee joint. Scand J Rheumatol 1983;12:152–6.

[61] Hurley MV, Scott DL, Rees J, Newham DJ. Sensorimotor changes and functional performance in patients with knee osteoarthritis. Ann Rheum Dis 1997;56:641–8.

[62] Sharma L, Pai YC, Holtkamp K, Rymer WZ. Is knee joint proprioception worse in the arthritic knee versus the unaffected knee in unilateral knee osteoarthritis? Arthritis Rheum 1997;40: 1518–25.

[63] Ekdaho C, Andersson S, Moritz U, Svensson B. Dynamic versus statis training in patients with rheumatoid arthritis. Scand J Rheum 1990;19:17–26.

[64] Minor M, Hewett J, Webel R, Anderson S, Kay D. Efficacy of physical conditioning exercise in patients with rheumatoid arthritis and osteoarthritis. Athritis Rheum 1989;32:1396–405.

[65] Rogind H, Bibow-Nielsen B, Jensen B, Moller HC, Frimodt-Moller H, Bliddal H. The effects of a physical training program on patients with osteoarthritis of the knees. Arch Phys Med Rehabil 1998;79:1421–7.

[66] Peterson M, Kovar-Toledano PA, Otis JC, Allegrante JP, Mackenzie CR, Gutin B, et al. Effect of a walking program on gait characteristics in patients with osteoarthritis. Arthritis Care Res 1993;6:11–6.

[67] Kerrigan DC, Lelas JL, Goggins J, Merriman GJ, Kaplan RJ, Felson DT. Effectiveness of a lateral-wedge insole on knee varus torque in patients with knee osteoarthritis. Arch Phys Med Rehabil 2002;83:889–93.

[68] Pollo FE, Otis JC, Backus SI, Warren RF, Wickiewicz TL. Reduction of medial compartment loads with valgus bracing of the osteoarthritic knee. Am J Sports Med 2002;30:414–21.

[69] Voloshin A, Wosk J. Influence of artificial shock absorbers on human gait. Clin Orthop 1981;52–6.

[70] Kerrigan DC, Lelas JL, Karvosky ME. Women's shoes and knee osteoarthritis. Lancet 2001; 357:1097–8.

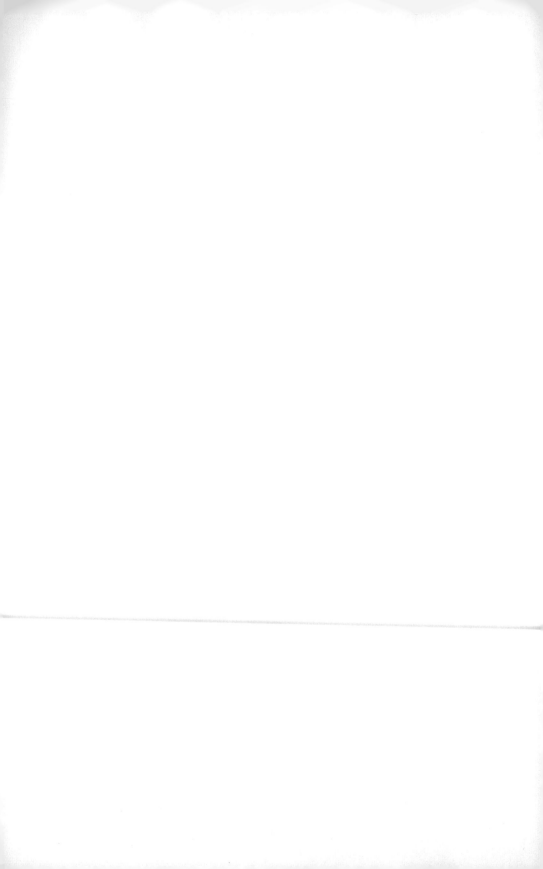

ELSEVIER
SAUNDERS

Clin Sports Med 24 (2005) 133–152

CLINICS
IN SPORTS
MEDICINE

The Use of Arthroscopy in the Athlete with Knee Osteoarthritis

George T. Calvert, MD, Rick W. Wright, MD*

Department of Orthopaedic Surgery, Washington University School of Medicine, Campus Box 8233, St. Louis, MO 63110, USA

The use of arthroscopy in the classification, diagnosis, and treatment of knee osteoarthritis (OA) is currently a source of considerable debate among sports medicine practitioners as well as the general medical community [1–10]. No consensus guidelines for when or how to use arthroscopy in the treatment of OA have been developed. This article summarizes the current evidence regarding the use of arthroscopy in knee OA. Data from the most recent articles, European publications, and the rheumatology literature has been included. The author's current treatment algorithm for the athlete with OA is presented.

Arthroscopic classification

Multiple classification systems for assessing articular cartilage lesions have been developed [11–16] (Table 1). Of particular interest to the arthroscopist, many of the commonly used systems were developed at open arthrotomy [11–13] or cadaver dissection [14], and several systems were designed for evaluation of the patella alone [11–13]. The commonly used system of Outerbridge [11] was developed based upon incidental observation of patellar articular cartilage defects in 196 cases of open medial meniscectomy. The more recently developed classifications of Noyes [15] and the French Society of Arthroscopists (SFA) [16] were created specifically for arthroscopic assessment of the entire knee.

Little has been published on the validity, accuracy, and reliability of the arthroscopic classifications [16–19]. Validity describes how well a system actu-

---

* Corresponding author.

E-mail address: wrightr@wustl.edu (R.W. Wright).

Table 1
Arthroscopic classifications

System (date)	Source	Area	Surface description	Depth/extent	Diameter
Outerbridge (1961)	Arthrotomy	Patella	I. Softening and swelling II. Fragmentation and fissuring III. Fragmentation and fissuring IV. Erosion to bone		II. <1/2 inch III. >1/2 inch
Bentley (1970)	Arthrotomy	Patella	I. Fibrillation or fissure II. Fibrillation or fissure III. Fibrillation or fissure IV. Fibrillation +/− exposed bone		I. <0.5 cm II. 0.5–1.0 cm III. 1.0–2.0 cm IV. >2.0 cm
Insall (1976)	Arthrotomy	Patella	I. Swelling and softening II. Deep fissures III. Fibrillation IV. Exposed bone		
Casscells (1978)	Cadaver	Knee	I. Superficial involvement II. Deeper involvement III. Exposed bone IV. Complete loss cartilage		I. <1 cm II. 1–2 cm III. 2–4 cm IV. Extensive
Noyes (1989)	Arthoscopy	Knee	I. Surface intact II. Surface damaged III. Bone exposed	A. Resilient B. Deformed A. <1/2 thickness B. >1/2 thickness A. Bone intact B. Bone cavitation	<10 mm <15 mm <20 mm <25 mm >25 mm
SFA (1994)	Arthoscopy	Knee	I. Softening and swelling II. Superficial fissuring III. Deep fissuring IV. Exposed bone	% surface area involvement	

ally measures what it purports to measure. The SFA group provided internal and external validation data for their system [16]. They first showed correlation between visual analog scale scoring of the arthroscopist's overall assessment of cartilage damage with the surface characteristics and depth of the lesions (intrinsic validity). Patient age and extent of radiographic changes were also correlated (extrinsic validity). The SFA grading system (Table 1) was then validated using the visual analog scale in a multicenter study of 755 knee arthroscopy cases. Accuracy is the degree to which a measurement represents the true value of the attribute being measured. This can be determined only if a "gold standard" reference value is accepted. Cameron et al [19] used postarthroscopy dissection of cadaver knees in their determination of the accuracy of the Outerbridge classification. They found an accuracy of 68% among nine orthopedic surgeons with decreasing accuracy for low-grade lesions.

Reliability of a classification is often quantified by the kappa coefficient, which represents the agreement among observers not attributable to chance alone. A value of 1 represents perfect agreement, whereas a value of 0 represents agreement expected from chance alone. The three publications reporting intraobserver and interobserver reliability kappa coefficients demonstrated a wide range of values (Table 2). All are limited by use of arthroscopy videos, which do not provide tactile feedback. Overall, intraobserver reliability is better than interobserver reliability. Training in the application of the system [17] and surgeon experience [19] can improve reliability.

Diagnostic arthroscopy

Accurate diagnosis of the athlete with knee pain can be challenging. After history and physical examination, radiography remains the initial diagnostic study for most practitioners. Several authors have studied the correlation between arthroscopic and radiographic findings [20–25]. Using arthroscopic exam as the gold standard, the sensitivity, specificity, positive predictive value, and negative predictive value of radiographs can be calculated (Table 3). Sensitivity and specificity were found to range from 0.02 [25] to 0.91 [24] and 0.61 [22] to 1.00 [21], respectively. This variation represents differences in patient characteristics (age, sex ratio, symptom duration), site studied (medial compartment, lateral compartment), and radiographic technique (anterior/posterior [AP] extension, posterior/anterior [PA] flexed). The authors also used different radiographic and arthroscopic classifications. Studies of older patients and those with known degenerative arthritis [21,24] show higher sensitivity and specificity than studies of younger sports medicine clinic patients [22,25]. Overall, the studies indicate that radiographs have higher specificity, identifying patients who do not have arthritis, than sensitivity, identifying patients who do have arthritis. Correspondingly, radiographs have a low false positive rate but a high false negative rate.

Comparison of magnetic resonance imaging (MRI) and arthroscopy has also been performed [26–28]. Sensitivity has ranged from 0.31 [26] to 0.87 [28].

Table 2
Reliability of arthroscopic classification systems

Author	Brismar	Cameron	Cameron	Brismar	Ayral	Ayral
Date	2002	2003	2003	2002	1998	1998
Classification	Outerbridge	Outerbridge	Outerbridge	SFA	SFA	SFA
Observers	4	9	2	4	9	9
Surgeries	19	6	6	19	5	5
Note			>5-yr experience		Pretraining	Posttraining
Intraobserver reliability	0.42–0.66	0.8	0.91	0.50–0.61		
Interobserver reliability	0.47	0.52	0.72	0.49	0.44	0.87

Table 3
Radiographic diagnosis of arthroscopically confirmed OA

Author	Wright	Wright	Wright	Wright	Rosenberg	Rosenberg
Compartment	Medial	Medial	Lateral	Lateral	Medial	Medial
X-ray technique	AP Extension	PA Flexed	AP extension	PA flexed	AP extension	PA flexed
Patient age	38 (12–85)	38 (12–85)	38 (12–85)	38 (12–85)	N/R	N/R
Symptom duration	any	any	any	any	>6 months	>6 months
Classification	Outerbridge	Outerbridge	Outerbridge	Outerbridge	Outerbridge	Outerbridge
Sensitivity	0.03	0.05	0.11	0.02	0.25	0.86
Specificity	0.98	0.99	0.92	0.95	0.96	1
PPV	0.57	0.87	0.31	0.14	0.88	1
NPV	0.59	0.6	0.77	0.76	0.55	0.87

Author	Rosenberg	Rosenberg	Fife	Fife	Brandt	Wada	Lysholm
Compartment	Lateral	Lateral	Medial	Lateral	All	Medial	All
X-ray technique	AP extension	PA flexed	AP extension	AP extension	AP extension	AP extension	N/R
Patient age	N/R	N/R	36.4 (12–69)	36.4 (12–69)	40.6 (14–69)	65.2 (41–84)	50.7 (26–70)
Symptom duration	>6 months	>6 months	chronic	chronic	>2 months	>3 months	<12 months
Classification	Outerbridge	Outerbridge	Bentley	Bentley	Outerbridge	Koshino	Outerbridge
Sensitivity	0.3	0.8	0.67	0.27	N/R	0.91	N/R
Specificity	0.96	1	0.61	0.9	N/R	0.73	N/R
PPV	0.6	1	0.42	0.41	N/R	0.98	N/R
NPV	0.86	0.96	0.87	0.89	N/R	0.41	N/R

Abbreviation: N/R, not reported.

Again, differences in patient characteristics, imaging techniques, and classification schemes likely explain much of the difference. MRI interpretation is also more difficult and thus susceptible to interobserver variation based upon experience and training. Similar to radiographs, MRI generally has higher specificity than sensitivity.

As indicated by the above discussion, arthroscopy remains the gold standard for diagnosis of articular cartilage lesions. Like all diagnostic tools, its use depends on the individual clinical situation and the index of suspicion of the clinician. Advantages in comparison to noninvasive imaging include direct visualization, tactile feedback, and ability to simultaneously provide treatment. Disadvantages include the risk associated with invasive procedure and cost.

Arthroscopic lavage

The oldest and simplest arthroscopic treatment of OA is lavage. Burman reported symptomatic relief in a series of 30 patients in 1934 [29]. Subsequently, numerous studies have evaluated lavage alone [30,31], lavage in combination with other treatments [32,33], and lavage in comparison with other treatments [34–41]. Differences in surgical techniques, patient populations, outcome measures, and statistical analyses have resulted in variable findings. Consequently, different recommendations have been made. Despite this, some general principles are evident. All studies show improvement after lavage in comparison to preoperative pain and function. The reason for improvement is unknown. The amount of improvement, percentage of patients improved, and duration of improvement varies between studies.

Surgical technique can vary by the amount of irrigation fluid and the mode of delivery. Dawes et al performed an observer-blinded, randomized controlled trial comparing needle lavage of 2 L saline with injection of 10 mL saline in 20 patients [35]. Although both groups showed improvement in pain and function, the only significant difference between groups was decreased thigh circumference in the lavage group at 12 weeks. The power of this study to prove equivalence was obviously limited by sample size. Kalunian et al performed a double-blind randomized controlled trial comparing visually guided needle irrigation with 3 L and 250 mL. Neither intervention generated a statistically significant improvement in overall outcome as judged by Western Ontario and McMaster University Osteoarthritis Index (WOMAC) at 12 months. However, the 3-L lavage group did have statistically significant improvement in the WOMAC pain subscale and visual analog pain scale (VAS) at 12 months. Chang et al performed an observer blind randomized controlled trial comparing arthroscopic debridement with office-based needle lavage with 1-L saline in 32 patients. Differences in technique included lavage versus debridement and needle irrigation versus formal arthroscopy. No differences between groups were found at 3 months or 1 year. Again, sample size limits the ability to assess equivalence between groups.

Arthroscopic lavage and conservative medical management have been compared. Livesley et al performed a nonrandomized, nonblinded prospective study comparing 37 patients receiving lavage and physical therapy with 24 patients receiving physical therapy alone [36]. Both groups displayed improvement in pain and physical signs of knee irritation. The lavage group showed greater and longer lasting improvement. A double-blind randomized placebo-controlled trial of arthroscopy plus corticosteroid injection versus arthroscopy plus placebo injection in 71 patients was recently published [33]. The corticosteroid group showed statistically significant greater response to therapy on the Osteoarthritis Research Society International criteria than placebo at 4 weeks. No differences were noted at greater than 4 weeks. Ravaud et al performed a multicenter randomized controlled trial comparing needle arthroscopic lavage plus corticosteroid injection, needle arthroscopic lavage alone, corticosteroid alone, and placebo injection in 98 patients [32]. The trial was double blind for injection but open for arthroscopy. Lavage improved VAS pain scale up to the trial endpoint of 24 weeks. Corticosteroid injection improved VAS pain scale only at weeks 1 and 4. The combination lavage plus injection group showed an additive but not synergistic response of the two treatments.

Arthroscopic lavage and arthroscopic debridement have been compared in multiple studies [34,37–41]. Study design, patient characteristics, and study results are summarized in Table 4. Overall, two studies demonstrated increased benefit with debridement [34,39] and three studies failed to show major differences between interventions [37,38,41]. The two studies favoring debridement have design characteristics worthy of specific mention. The study of Jackson et al was retrospective, and therefore susceptible to selection bias. The

Table 4
Comparison studies of lavage and debridement

Author	Jackson	Gibson	Chang	Hubbard	Moseley
Date	1986	1992	1993	1996	2002
Study design	RCT	PRCT	PRCT	PRCT	PRCT
Total patients	207	20	32	76	180
Follow-up (months)	39.6	12	12	54	24
Percent withdrawal	20%	0	0	24%	8%
Lavage group	53	10	14	36	61
debridement group	113	10	18	40	59
Age lavage	N/R	53 +/− 10 (38–68)	65 +/− 13	N/R	51.2 +/− 10.5
Age debridement	N/A	57 +/− 7(45–69)	61 +/− 11	N/R	53.6 +/− 12.2
Sex lavage M/F	N/R	6/4	4/10	N/R	54/7
Sex debridement M/F	N/A	8/2	5/13	N/R	57/2
Symptom lavage (month)	N/R	120+/−108	51	>12	>6
Symptom control (month)	N/A	96+/−84	53	>12	>6
Blind assessor	N/A	N/R	Yes	No	Yes
% Good/excellent lavage	45%	N/R	58%	12%	N/R
% Good/excellent debridement	68%	N/R	44%	59%	N/R

Abbreviations: N/A, not applicable; N/R, not reported; PRCT, prospective randomized controlled trial; RCT, retrospective control trial.

Table 5
Arthroscopic debridement case series

Author	Sprague	Salisbury	Baumgaertner	Timoney	McLaren	Gross	Aichroth	Olgilvie-Harris
Date	1981	1985	1990	1990	1991	1991	1991	1991
Study design	RCS	RCS	RCS	RCS	RCS	RCS	PCS	RCS
Total patients	72	41	44	108	170	40	280	441
Total knees	78	48	49	111	170	43	280	441
Follow-up (months)	13.6	27.5	33	50.6	25	24	44	48
Withdrawal	12%	21%	7%	8%	N/R	20%	9%	20%
Age	56 (24–78)	N/R	63 (51–76)	58.1 (40–81)	54 (23–82)	54 (40–71)	49 (28–82)	58 (28–92)
Sex M/F	45/27	N/R	N/R	75/33	119/51	28/22	184/70	N/R
Symptoms (month)	N/R	N/R	all > 6	avg 48.9	N/R	all > 6	N/R	N/R
Outcome device	Author's	Author's	Author's	HSS	Author's	HSS	Author's	Author's
Assessor	Surgeon	Surgeon	Surgeon	Surgeon	Surgeon	Surgeon	Physician	Surgeon
Follow-up method	phone	clinic	clinic	phone	mail	clinic	clinic	clinic
Xrays > 50% JSN	N/R	N/R	> 90%	N/R	N/R	4.70%	39%	N/R
% Outerbridge 4	61%	N/R	> 80%	> 50%	N/R	N/R	26%	37%
% Good/excellent	74%	N/R	40%	45%	65%	72.10%	75%	53%
% Meniscus tear	81%	N/R	84%	> 75%	N/R	70%	81%	35% unstable
% Further surgery	N/R	N/R	29%	N/R	12.40%	N/R	14%	N/R

Author	Yang	Harwin	McGinley	Shannon	Bohnsack	Fond	Jackson	Dervin
Date	1995	1999	1999	2001	2002	2002	2003	2003
Study design	RCS	RCS	RCS	RCS	RCS	RCS	RCS	PCS
Total patients	103	190	77	54	104	36	121	126
Total knees	105	204	91	55	104	36	121	126
Follow-up (months)	11.7	88.8	158.4	29.6	64.8	60	48–72	24
Withdrawal	N/R	14%	52%	N/R	N/R	44%	2.50%	19.20%
Age	64.2 (60–81)	62.1 (32–88)	62.6 (55–82)	60.9 (48–83)	60 (50–83)	64.8 (50–82)	56.4 (22–85)	61.7 (43–75)
Sex M/F	83/20	81/109	N/R	24/30	50/54	N/R	N/R	59/67
Symptoms (month)	82% > 1mo	N/R	N/R	37% > 1 yr	N/R	60	N/R	N/R
Outcome device	Author's	Author's	Tegner	Duke	Lysholm	HSS	Author's	SF-36, WOMAC
Assessor	Surgeon	Surgeon	Surgeon	Surgeon	Surgeon	Surgeon	Surgeon	Patient
Follow-up method	N/R	N/R	Phone	Phone	N/R	Clinic	Clinic	Mail
X-rays > 50% JSN	N/R	N/R	100%	N/R	100%	N/R	N/R	N/R
% Outerbridge 4	N/R	N/R	N/R	N/R	N/R	N/R	N/R	> 30%
% Good/excellent	64.80%	63.20%	N/R	48%	65%	69.40%	50.40%	44%
% Meniscus tear	96%	N/R	N/R	22% treated	> 82%	94.40%	52.10%	63% unstable
% Further surgery	4.80%	26.50%	37%	25.90%	20%	22%	28.90%	N/R

Abbreviations: avg, average; N/R, Not reported; PCS, Prospective case series; RCS, Retrospective case series; yr, year.

study of Hubbard, although prospective and randomized, had the nonblinded operating surgeon as the sole assessor of outcome. The studies demonstrating equivalence also have design issues. The trials of Gibson et al and Chang et al had 20 and 32 patients, respectively. Small sample size increases the possibility of beta error or failure to reject the null hypothesis thus assuming equivalence when, in fact, there is a difference. Comparison between lavage and debridement in the study by Moseley et al may have been biased by resection of bucket handle meniscus tears in the lavage group. If the two techniques are truly equivalent, as three of the studies mentioned above suggest, then lavage may offer considerable advantages in convenience and cost. Needle lavage can be performed in an office setting with local anesthesia. The cost of office based lavage was $3480 less than operative arthroscopy in the study of Chang et al.

Arthroscopic debridement

Data from 16 case series reporting on arthroscopic debridement of OA are reviewed in Table 5 [42–57]. Good and excellent results, as defined by the respective authors, are reported in 40% to 75% of patients at final follow-up. Patient characteristics associated with positive outcomes in multiple studies include less severe disease at the time of surgery, acute symptoms, normal lower extremity alignment, mechanical symptoms, and surgically treatable meniscus lesions. Conversely, severe disease, chronic symptoms, varus or valgus defor-mity, lack of discrete intraarticular pathology, and history of prior surgery cor-relate with poorer outcome in many studies. Results of debridement deteriorate with time. This is evident both within individual studies [45,49,55,56] and in comparison of studies with short-term follow-up [42] to those with intermediate-term follow-up [51].

Variability in patient outcomes among studies of debridement is multifactorial. Different patient populations, outcome tools, follow-up protocols, and statistical analyses were used. By definition, none of the case series used a control group. Many series report results on fewer than 100 patients [42–44,47,52,53,55], introducing the possibility of sampling error. Loss to follow-up was over 40% in two studies [52,55] and not reported in four others [46,50,53,54]. Although average age was 49 or older in all studies, the age ranges were quite variable with some studies including 20- to 40-year-old patients and others excluding all patients below fifty (Table 5). It is questionable whether OA in a 25-year-old is the same entity as in a 75-year-old even if both meet American College of Rheumatology (ACR) criteria. In the series of Baumgaertner et al, 8% of the patients have rheumatoid arthritis [44]. Although OA of the knee has a female predominance, only 3 of 16 studies listed in Table 5 included more women than men. Only two studies listed someone other than the operating surgeon as the primary assessor of outcome [48,57]. A clinician other the operating surgeon interviewed and examined all patients in the study of Aichroth et al. Whether the evaluating clinician was blinded to the findings of surgery was not reported. The study of Devin et al used validated patient-reported quality-of-life indices. Follow-up data collection also varied between case series. Four studies used phone interviews [42,45,52,53], and two series used mailed surveys [46,57].

Arthroscopic debridement has been compared with medical management in at least one prospective trial [58]. Eighty consecutive patients over age 50 were randomized to surgery or medical management. Age, sex ratio, and disease severity were similar between groups. Medical management consisted of nonsteroidal antiinflammatory drugs (NSAIDs) and activity modification. All patients received comparable physical therapy. The Hospital for Special Surgery Knee Rating Score was used to assess outcome. Operated patients had statistically significant greater improvement at final follow-up. At 3-year follow-up 67% of operated patients were improved and 45% of medically treated patients were improved. Use of NSAIDs in the operative group and use of corticosteroid injections in either group was not reported.

Simultaneous comparison of lavage, debridement, and sham surgery was reported in the previously mentioned trial of Moseley et al (Table 4). This and the pilot study that preceded it are the only reports in the literature including an operative placebo control group [40,41]. The trial showed significant improvement in pain and function in the three groups, and failed to show any difference in outcome among the three groups. Strengths of study include prospective analysis, randomization, single surgeon, double-blind analysis, low withdrawal, and use of validated patient-reported outcome measures. The treatment groups had similar age, sex ratio, symptoms, and radiographic disease severity. Extrapolation from this study of a predominantly male Veteran's Administration patient population to the general population has been questioned. Also, 44% of eligible patients refused to participate introducing the possibility of selection bias. Although validated outcome instruments including the Short Form 36 and Arthritis Impact Measurement Scales were used, the primary outcome scale was nonvalidated and created for the study. Even if the criticisms of equivalence between treatment groups are accepted, the dramatic response of patients to placebo surgery remains. When patients were questioned as to which procedure had been performed, they answered no more frequently than they would by chance alone.

All of the preceding studies report data from selected surgeons publishing in academic journals. Use of arthroscopic debridement in the province of Ontario between 1992 and 1996 has been reported [59]. This is the only population research available. On average, 1.4 arthroscopic debridements were performed per 1000 residents. The complication rate was 1.9%. At 3-year follow-up, 2.9% underwent high tibial osteotomy, 7.7% underwent repeat arthroscopy, and 18.4% underwent total knee arthroplasty (TKA). Thirty-three percent over age 70 underwent TKA. Geographic regions within the province in which the rate of debridement was higher than average, and also had higher rates of subsequent TKA among patients over 70. This suggests overuse of the procedure in elderly patients in some areas.

Abrasion arthroplasty and microfracture

Arthroscopic techniques to produce cartilage regeneration in the knee by mechanical stimulation were introduced by Johnson in 1981 [60]. His original technique involved intracortical debridement of 1-2 mm of sclerotic bone with a motorized bur. Simultaneous, standard lavage and debridement is performed. This is followed by 2 months nonweight-bearing activity. He reported a series of 104 patients in whom 75% reported improvement at 2 years (Table 6). Only seven reoperations were performed. Friedman et al reported a higher rate of improvement after abrasion arthroplasty compared with debridement at 12-month follow-up examination [61]. Two subsequent retrospective case–control series have reported worse results and higher reoperation rates with abrasion arthroplasty compared with standard debridement [62,63] (Table 6). The most striking finding in these studies is 54% rate of total knee arthroplasty within 4 years in the study of Rand et al (Table 6). Subsequent debate has ensued with some supporting continued use of the technique [64], and others refuting its efficacy [6,10,65]. In light of the susceptibility of retrospective trials and series to selection bias and the known placebo response to arthroscopic treatment of knee OA, prospective randomized controlled trials will be needed to definitively resolve the debate.

Arthroscopic bone drilling [66] and microfracture [67] have also been used to treat knee OA. The theoretic advantage of microfracture with an arthroscopic awl is generation of less heat necrosis than motorized drilling or burring. Drilling

Table 6
Abrasion arthroplasty studies

Author	Friedman	Johnson	Bert	Rand
Date	1984	1986	1989	1991
Study design	RCT	RCS	RCT	RCT
Abrasion patients	41	95 (99 knees)	59	28
Debridement patients	37	N/A	67	28
Follow-up abrasion (months)	12	>24	60	45.6
Follow-up debridement (months)	12	N/A	60	48
Follow-up loss abrasion	N/R	9%	9%	18%
Follow-up loss debridement	N/R	N/A	9%	N/R
Age abrasion	54 (N/R)	60 (29–88)	66 (46–84)	63 (45–76)
Age debridement	57 (29–71)	N/A	61 (39–82)	60 (45–79)
Sex Abrasion M/F	N/R	59/45	58% M	18/10
Sex debridement M/F	28/9	N/A	54% M	18/10
Outcome	Author's	Author's	Author's/HSS	Author's/HSS
Blind assesor	No	No	No	No
% Good/excellent abrasion	53%	75%	51%	39%
% Good/excellent debridement	32%	N/A	66%	79%
Non-weight bearing (weeks)	3–4 wk	8 wk	6 wk	8 wk
% Further surgery abrasion	N/R	8%	20%	54%
% Further surgery debridement	N/R	N/A	15%	11%

Abbreviations: N/A, not applicable; N/R, not reported; RCS, retrospective case series; RCT, retrospective control trial.

in 77 knees of 73 patient has been compared with an age-matched control group of 16 arthroscopic lavage patients [66]. Relief of pain was reported in 69% of drilling patients and 19% of lavage patients. Steadman et al report 75% of patients in their series had improved pain at 3- to 5-year follow-up. Again, prospective randomized controlled trials will be needed to assess benefit of these procedures in comparison to lavage, debridement, and placebo.

Partial meniscectomy in patients with osteoarthritis

Meniscus tears are common among patients with OA. Series of arthroscopic debridement report rates ranging between 22% and 94% (Table 5). Multiple authors have studied arthroscopic partial meniscectomy in knees with OA [68–72]. Study characteristic and results are reviewed in Table 7. Patients with meniscus tears and associated OA achieved benefit from arthroscopic surgery across studies. However, rate of good and excellent results, based on the author's criteria, were consistently lower than among patients treated for meniscus tear without associated OA. Reoperation rates were also higher among patients with associated OA. Longer duration of symptoms [68,72] and radiographic evidence

Table 7
Arthrospic meniscectomy and OA

Author	Jackson	Rand	Bonamo	Matsusue
Date	1982	1985	1992	1996
Study design	RCT	RCS	RCT	RCT
OA + meniscus tear (MT)	47 (51 knees)	84 (87 knees)	63	15 knees
Meniscus tear (MT)	19 (20 knees)	N/A	118	53 knees
Follow-up (months) OA + MT	30	24	39.6	93.6
Follow-up (months) MT	30	N/A	42	93.6
Withdrawal OA + MT	3%	9%	N/R	N/R
Withdrawal MT	3%	N/A	N/R	N/R
Age OA + MT	55.3	62 (29–84)	57 (40–77)	51.5
Age MT	50.2	N/A	50 (40–78)	48.7
Sex M/F OA + MT	35/12	47/37	78/40	N/R
Sex M/F MT	18/1	N/A	48/15	N/R
Sx (month) OA + MT	15.7	N/R	64% > 6 months	65
Sx (month) MT	6.3	N/A	52% > 6 months	35
Assessor	Surgeon	Surgeon	Surgeon	Surgeon
Outcome device	Author's	Author's	Author's	Author's
Fellow-up method	Clinical exam	Mail	Clinical exam	Clinical exam
% Good/excellent OA + MT	80%	84%	83%	47%
% Good/excellent MT	95%	N/A	94%	94%
% Mechanical Sx OA + MT	30%	48–74%	N/R	N/R
% Mechanical Sx MT	35%	N/A	N/R	N/R
% Further surgery OA + MT	9%	7%	4.20%	N/R
% Further surgery MT	0.00%	N/A	1.50	N/R

Abbreviations: MT, meniscus tear; OA, osteoarthristis; RCS, retrospective case series; RCT, retrospective control trial; Sx, symptoms.

of degenerative disease [69] adversely affected outcome. Sex, age, and a history of precipitating trauma did not have significant prognostic value.

Recently, MRI evaluation of meniscus tears among patients older than 45 years with and without OA, as defined by ACR criteria, was studied [73]. Meniscus tear was defined as signal change extending to the articular surface. Comparison of 154 OA patients with 49 asymptomatic controls was made. Validated outcome measures were used (WOMAC and pain visual analog scale). Meniscus tears were common among patients with symptomatic OA (86%) and asymptomatic volunteers (67%). Prevalence of meniscus tears increased with increasing radiographic severity of OA. Individuals with severe radiographic change as graded by Kellgren-Lawrence criteria had a 100% rate of meniscus tear. Within the symptomatic OA group, there was no difference in pain or WOMAC score between those with and without meniscus tears. Limitations of the study include lack of arthroscopic confirmation of the MRI findings, lack of clinical symptomatology data (locking, catching), and difference in weight between the study groups. Despite these limitations, one can conclude that meniscus tears identifiable by MRI are extremely common among individuals over age 45. The role of meniscus tears in the causation of symptoms among patients with OA is called into question.

Anterior cruciate ligament reconstruction in the arthritic patient

Symptomatic knee instability combined with arthrosis in the active patient is a challenging combination. Arthroscopy can be used for diagnosis, debridement, and assistance with reconstruction. Short and intermediate term follow-up of arthritic patients treated with arthroscopically assisted or endoscopic anterior cruciate ligament (ACL) reconstruction reveals significant improvements in pain, stability, and function [74,75]. The authors of both studies counseled patients to avoid high-impact activities such as distance running and cutting sports. Shelbourne and Gray have reported retrospective objective follow-up of 482 patients at 7.6 years post-op and retrospective subjective follow-up of 928 patients at 8.6 years [76]. All patients underwent ACL reconstruction; status of the menisci and articular cartilage was noted at surgery. Patients with articular cartilage damage had lower subjective scores, lower modified International Knee Documentation Committee scores, and a higher rate of radiographic abnormalities. The authors concluded that in order of importance, articular cartilage damage, partial or total medial meniscectomy, and partial or total lateral meniscectomy adversely affect the outcome of ACL reconstruction.

Arthroscopy and high tibial osteotomy

Arthroscopy has been combined with high tibial osteotomy (HTO) for both diagnostic and therapeutic goals. Keene et al have evaluated short- [77] and intermediate-term [78] results of diagnostic arthroscopy combined with HTO. Arthroscopy failed to provide prognostic information in either study. Presence of bicompartmental and tricompartmental OA at arthroscopy did not predict worse outcome. Adequate valgus correction was the primary determinant of outcome in both studies. Other authors recommend routine arthroscopy before HTO [79,80]. They stress the low morbidity of the procedure and the ability to treat concomitant intraarticular pathology. Finally, operative indications and contraindications for HTO are not yet strictly defined. The use of diagnostic arthroscopy to exclude candidates remains undefined.

Arthroscopic debridement, drilling, and abrasion arthroplasty have been combined with HTO [79,81]. One prospective, nonrandomized, comparison trial has been performed [81]. Patients were evaluated by repeat arthroscopy at 1 year and Japanese Orthopaedic Association knee score at 4.8 years in the abrasion group and 3.5 years in the HTO only group. Repeat arthroscopy revealed statistically significant more fibrocartilage filling of articular surface defects in the abrasion plus HTO group. However, there were no differences in clinical outcome between groups. Schultz et al reported similar finding in a retrospective comparison of diagnostic arthroscopy, drilling, and abrasion arthroplasty in conjunction with HTO [79]. No difference in clinical outcome was found at 1-year follow-up.

Author's preferred method

A few data points are critical during the workup and evaluation of the patient considering arthroscopic treatment of their knee pain. During the physical examination and history we want to elicit any symptoms of mechanical locking or catching. In addition, joint line tenderness and a palpable clunk during a McMurray exam are valuable information. All patients evaluated in our clinics for knee pain either bring or undergo bilateral weight-bearing X-rays. We use the Rosenberg view, but either view is acceptable in a sports medicine clinic.

If the patient has a history and physical examination consistent with a meniscal tear and no joint space narrowing is noted on standing X-rays then we will discuss obtaining an MRI to verify the diagnosis. If the patient has classic locking symptoms and does not desire to undergo an MRI, then we will discuss proceeding with arthroscopic evaluation. If the patient has joint space narrowing on weight-bearing X-rays then we typically begin treatment by maximizing conservative management of their arthritis. This includes recommending NSAIDs, ice, and physical therapy especially for anterior knee pain symptoms. If this fails to control their symptoms, then we will discuss corticosteroid or hyaluronic acid injections. Alignment X-rays to include the hip, knee, and ankle for consideration of an osteotomy will be obtained at this time.

Patients with normal alignment and greater than 50% joint space remaining who undergo corticosteroid or hyaluronic acid injections with quick return of their pain in less than a month following injection are counseled regarding arthroscopic debridement as a treatment option. This is especially true if they have continuing mechanical symptoms and joint line tenderness. If they obtain several months relief following injection then we believe that the majority of their symptoms can be controlled with conservative measures. Patients considering arthroscopic debridement are counseled regarding potential benefit and the fact that the procedure will not be curative.

At the time of arthroscopy all meniscal tears are debrided. Chondral flaps and loose articular cartilage are debrided with mechanical shavers and biters. If there are focal areas of complete articular cartilage loss surrounded by relatively normal articular cartilage the patient may be a candidate for microfracture. If the articular cartilage wear is diffuse throughout the compartment or entire knee, then simple debridement is performed. We do not inject the knee with corticosteroids at the time of arthroscopy, to avoid any increased chance of infection. Following arthroscopy, the patients undergo routine postoperative management with physical therapy for range of motion and strengthening and ice therapy to minimize swelling. Patients that undergo microfracture are nonweight bearing for the initial 6 weeks.

Summary

Arthroscopy is an important technique in the diagnosis, classification, and treatment of the athlete with OA. Reliability of the current classification systems improves with training and experience. Arthroscopy remains superior to imaging in the diagnosis of OA. Arthroscopic lavage and debridement provide benefit in a significant percentage of patients. The reasons for improvement are not fully defined. Arthroscopic treatment of OA is not curative, and results deteriorate with time. Variability in the use of medical management, arthroscopy, osteotomy, and arthroplasty remains among different practitioners. Indications for arthroscopy require further clarification based upon empiric evidence.

References

[1] Jackson RW. The role of arthroscopy in the management of the arthritic knee. Clin Orthop 1974; 101(1):28–35.
[2] Schonholtz GJ. Arthroscopic debridement of the knee joint. Orthop Clin North Am 1989;20(2): 257–63.
[3] Burks RT. Arthroscopy and degenerative arthritis of the knee: a review of the literature. Arthroscopy 1990;6(1):43–7.
[4] Ike RW. The role of arthroscopy in the differential diagnosis of osteoarthritis of the knee. Rheum Dis Clin North Am 1993;19(3):673–96.
[5] Novak PJ, Bach Jr BR. Selection criteria for knee arthroscopy in the osteoarthritic patient. Orthop Rev 1993;22(7):798–804.
[6] Jackson RW, Gilbert JE, Sharkey PF. Arthroscopic debridement versus arthroplasty in the osteoarthritic knee. J Arthroplasty 1997;12(4):465–9 [discussion 469–70].
[7] Goldman RT, Scuderi GR, Kelly MA. Arthroscopic treatment of the degenerative knee in older athletes. Clin Sports Med 1997;16(1):51–68.

[8] Buckwalter JA, Lane NE. Athletics and osteoarthritis. Am J Sports Med 1997;25(6):873–81.
[9] Hanssen AD, Stuart MJ, Scott RD, Scuderi GR. Surgical options for the middle-aged patient with osteoarthritis of the knee joint. Instr Course Lect 2001;50:499–511.
[10] Hunt SA, Jazrawi LM, Sherman OH. Arthroscopic management of osteoarthritis of the knee. J Am Acad Orthop Surg 2002;10(5):356–63.
[11] Outerbridge RE. The etiology of chondromalacia patellae. J Bone Joint Surg Br 1961;43-B: 752–7.
[12] Bentley G, Dowd G. Current concepts of etiology and treatment of chondromalacia patellae. Clin Orthop 1984;189:209–28.
[13] Insall J, Falvo KA, Wise DW. Chondromalacia Patellae. A prospective study. J Bone Joint Surg Am 1976;58(1):1–8.
[14] Casscells SW. Gross pathological changes in the knee joint of the aged individual: a study of 300 cases. Clin Orthop 1978;132:225–32.
[15] Noyes FR, Stabler CL. A system for grading articular cartilage lesions at arthroscopy. Am J Sports Med 1989;17(4):505–13.
[16] Dougados M, Ayral X, Listrat V, Gueguen A, Bahuaud J, Beaufils P, et al. The SFA system for assessing articular cartilage lesions at arthroscopy of the knee. Arthroscopy 1994;10(1):69–77.
[17] Ayral X, Gueguen A, Ike RW, Bonvarlet JP, Frizziero L, Kalunian K, et al. Inter-observer reliability of the arthroscopic quantification of chondropathy of the knee. Osteoarthritis Cartilage 1998;6(3):160–6.
[18] Brismar BH, Wredmark T, Movin T, Leandersson J, Svensson O. Observer reliability in the arthroscopic classification of osteoarthritis of the knee. J Bone Joint Surg Br 2002;84(1):42–7.
[19] Cameron ML, Briggs KK, Steadman JR. Reproducibility and reliability of the outerbridge classification for grading chondral lesions of the knee arthroscopically. Am J Sports Med 2003; 31(1):83–6.
[20] Lysholm J, Hamberg P, Gillquist J. The correlation between osteoarthrosis as seen on radiographs and on arthroscopy. Arthroscopy 1987;3(3):161–5.
[21] Rosenberg TD, Paulos LE, Parker RD, Coward DB, Scott SM. The forty-five-degree posteroanterior flexion weight-bearing radiograph of the knee. J Bone Joint Surg Am 1988;70(10): 1479–83.
[22] Fife RS, Brandt KD, Braunstein EM, et al. Relationship between arthroscopic evidence of cartilage damage and radiographic evidence of joint space narrowing in early osteoarthritis of the knee. Arthritis Rheum 1991;34(4):377–82.
[23] Brandt KD, Fife RS, Braunstein EM, Katz B, Shelbourne KD, Kalasinski LA, et al. Radiographic grading of the severity of knee osteoarthritis: relation of the Kellgren and Lawrence grade to a grade based on joint space narrowing, and correlation with arthroscopic evidence of articular cartilage degeneration. Arthritis Rheum 1991;34(11):1381–6.
[24] Wada M, Baba H, Imura S, Morita A, Kusaka Y. Relationship between radiographic classification and arthroscopic findings of articular cartilage lesions in osteoarthritis of the knee. Clin Exp Rheumatol 1998;16(1):15–20.
[25] Wright RW, Spindler KP, Boyce RH, Michener T, Shyr Y, McCarty EC. The sensitivity and specificity of standing knee radiographs (AP vs. PA flexion) in arthroscopically confirmed early arthritis. Clin Orthop, in press.
[26] Speer KP, Spritzer CE, Goldner JL, Garrett Jr WE. Magnetic resonance imaging of traumatic knee articular cartilage injuries. Am J Sports Med 1991;19(4):396–402.
[27] Broderick LS, Turner DA, Renfrew DL, Schnitzer TJ, Huff JP, Harris C. Severity of articular cartilage abnormality in patients with osteoarthritis: evaluation with fast spin-echo MR vs arthroscopy. AJR Am J Roentgenol 1994;162(1):99–103.
[28] Potter HG, Linklater JM, Allen AA, Hannafin JA, Haas SB. Magnetic resonance imaging of articular cartilage in the knee. An evaluation with use of fast-spin-echo imaging. J Bone Joint Surg Am 1998;80(9):1276–84.
[29] Burman MS. Arthroscopy or the direct visualization of joints: an experimental cadaver study. 1931. Clin Orthop 2001;390:5–9.

[30] Edelson R, Burks RT, Bloebaum RD. Short-term effects of knee washout for osteoarthritis. Am J Sports Med 1995;23(3):345–9.

[31] Kalunian KC, Moreland LW, Klashman DJ, Brion PH, Concoff AL, Myers S, et al. Visually-guided irrigation in patients with early knee osteoarthritis: a multicenter randomized, controlled trial. Osteoarthritis Cartilage 2000;8(6):412–8.

[32] Ravaud P, Moulinier L, Giraudeau B, Ayral X, Guerin C, Noel E, et al. Effects of joint lavage and steroid injection in patients with osteoarthritis of the knee: results of a multicenter, randomized, controlled trial. Arthritis Rheum 1999;42(3):475–82.

[33] Smith MD, Wetherall M, Darby T, Esterman A, Slavotinek J, Roberts-Thomson P, et al. A randomized placebo-controlled trial of arthroscopic lavage versus lavage plus intra-articular corticosteroids in the management of symptomatic osteoarthritis of the knee. Rheumatology (Oxford) 2003;42(12):1477–85.

[34] Jackson RW, Silver R, Marans H. Arthroscopic treatment of degenerative joint disease. Arthroscopy 1986;2(2):114.

[35] Dawes PT, Kirlew C, Haslock I. Saline washout for knee osteoarthritis: results of a controlled study. Clin Rheumatol 1987;6(1):61–3.

[36] Livesley PJ, Doherty M, Needoff M, Moulton A. Arthroscopic lavage of osteoarthritic knees. J Bone Joint Surg Br 1991;73(6):922–6.

[37] Gibson JN, White MD, Chapman VM, Strachan RK. Arthroscopic lavage and debridement for osteoarthritis of the knee. J Bone Joint Surg Br 1992;74(4):534–7.

[38] Chang RW, Falconer J, Stulberg SD, Arnold WJ, Manheim LM, Dyer AR. A randomized, controlled trial of arthroscopic surgery versus closed-needle joint lavage for patients with osteoarthritis of the knee. Arthritis Rheum 1993;36(3):289–96.

[39] Hubbard MJ. Articular debridement versus washout for degeneration of the medial femoral condyle. A five-year study. J Bone Joint Surg Br 1996;78(2):217–9.

[40] Moseley Jr JB, Wray NP, Kuykendall D, Willis K, Landon G. Arthroscopic treatment of osteoarthritis of the knee: a prospective, randomized, placebo-controlled trial. Results of a pilot study. Am J Sports Med 1996;24(1):28–34.

[41] Moseley JB, O'Malley K, Petersen NJ, Menke TJ, Brody BA, Kuykendall DH, et al. A controlled trial of arthroscopic surgery for osteoarthritis of the knee. N Engl J Med 2002;347(2):81–8.

[42] Sprague III NF. Arthroscopic debridement for degenerative knee joint disease. Clin Orthop 1981; 160:118–23.

[43] Salisbury RB, Nottage WM, Gardner V. The effect of alignment on results in arthroscopic debridement of the degenerative knee. Clin Orthop 1985;198:268–72.

[44] Baumgaertner MR, Cannon Jr WD, Vittori JM, Schmidt ES, Maurer RC. Arthroscopic debridement of the arthritic knee. Clin Orthop 1990;253:197–202.

[45] Timoney JM, Kneisl JS, Barrack RL, Alexander AH. Arthroscopy update #6. Arthroscopy in the osteoarthritic knee. Long-term follow-up. Orthop Rev 1990;19(4):371–3 [376–9].

[46] McLaren AC, Blokker CP, Fowler PJ, Roth JN, Rock MG. Arthroscopic debridement of the knee for osteoarthrosis. Can J Surg 1991;34(6):595–8.

[47] Gross DE, Brenner SL, Esformes I, Gross ML. Arthroscopic treatment of degenerative joint disease of the knee. Orthopedics 1991;14(12):1317–21.

[48] Aichroth PM, Patel DV, Moyes ST. A prospective review of arthroscopic debridement for degenerative joint disease of the knee. Int Orthop 1991;15(4):351–5.

[49] Ogilvie-Harris DJ, Fitsialos DP. Arthroscopic management of the degenerative knee. Arthroscopy 1991;7(2):151–7.

[50] Yang SS, Nisonson B. Arthroscopic surgery of the knee in the geriatric patient. Clin Orthop 1995;316:50–8.

[51] Harwin SF. Arthroscopic debridement for osteoarthritis of the knee: predictors of patient satisfaction. Arthroscopy 1999;15(2):142–6.

[52] McGinley BJ, Cushner FD, Scott WN. Debridement arthroscopy. 10-year followup. Clin Orthop 1999;367:190–4.

[53] Shannon FJ, Devitt AT, Poynton AR, Fitzpatrick P, Walsh MG. Short-term benefit of arthroscopic washout in degenerative arthritis of the knee. Int Orthop 2001;25(4):242–5.

[54] Bohnsack M, Lipka W, Ruhmann O, Peters G, Schmolke S, Wirth CJ. The value of knee arthroscopy in patients with severe radiological osteoarthritis. Arch Orthop Trauma Surg 2002; 122(8):451–3.

[55] Fond J, Rodin D, Ahmad S, Nirschl RP. Arthroscopic debridement for the treatment of osteoarthritis of the knee: 2- and 5-year results. Arthroscopy 2002;18(8):829–34.

[56] Jackson RW, Dieterichs C. The results of arthroscopic lavage and debridement of osteoarthritic knees based on the severity of degeneration: a 4- to 6-year symptomatic follow-up. Arthroscopy 2003;19(1):13–20.

[57] Dervin GF, Stiell IG, Rody K, Grabowski J. Effect of arthroscopic debridement for osteoarthritis of the knee on health-related quality of life. J Bone Joint Surg Am 2003;85-A(1):10–9.

[58] Merchan EC, Galindo E. Arthroscope-guided surgery versus nonoperative treatment for limited degenerative osteoarthritis of the femorotibial joint in patients over 50 years of age: a prospective comparative study. Arthroscopy 1993;9(6):663–7.

[59] Wai EK, Kreder HJ, Williams JI. Arthroscopic debridement of the knee for osteoarthritis in patients fifty years of age or older: utilization and outcomes in the Province of Ontario. J Bone Joint Surg Am 2002;84-A(1):17–22.

[60] Johnson LL. Arthroscopic abrasion arthroplasty historical and pathologic perspective: present status. Arthroscopy 1986;2(1):54–69.

[61] Friedman MJ, Berasi CC, Fox JM, Del Pizzo W, Snyder SJ, Ferkel RD. Preliminary results with abrasion arthroplasty in the osteoarthritic knee. Clin Orthop 1984;182:200–5.

[62] Bert JM, Maschka K. The arthroscopic treatment of unicompartmental gonarthrosis: a five-year follow-up study of abrasion arthroplasty plus arthroscopic debridement and arthroscopic debridement alone. Arthroscopy 1989;5(1):25–32.

[63] Rand JA. Role of arthroscopy in osteoarthritis of the knee. Arthroscopy 1991;7(4):358–63.

[64] Johnson LL. Arthroscopic abrasion arthroplasty: a review. Clin Orthop 2001;391(Suppl): S306–17.

[65] Bert JM. Role of abrasion arthroplasty and debridement in the management of osteoarthritis of the knee. Rheum Dis Clin North Am 1993;19(3):725–39.

[66] Pedersen MS, Moghaddam AZ, Bak K, Koch JS. The effect of bone drilling on pain in gonarthrosis. Int Orthop 1995;19(1):12–5.

[67] Steadman JR, Rodkey WG, Briggs KK. Microfracture to treat full-thickness chondral defects: surgical technique, rehabilitation, and outcomes. J Knee Surg 2002;15(3):170–6.

[68] Jackson RW, Rouse DW. The results of partial arthroscopic meniscectomy in patients over 40 years of age. J Bone Joint Surg Br 1982;64(4):481–5.

[69] Rand JA. Arthroscopic management of degenerative meniscus tears in patients with degenerative arthritis. Arthroscopy 1985;1(4):253–8.

[70] Bonamo JJ, Kessler KJ, Noah J. Arthroscopic meniscectomy in patients over the age of 40. Am J Sports Med 1992;20(4):422–8 [discussion 428–9].

[71] Rangger C, Klestil T, Gloetzer W, Kemmler G, Benedetto KP. Osteoarthritis after arthroscopic partial meniscectomy. Am J Sports Med 1995;23(2):240–4.

[72] Matsusue Y, Thomson NL. Arthroscopic partial medial meniscectomy in patients over 40 years old: a 5- to 11-year follow-up study. Arthroscopy 1996;12(1):39–44.

[73] Bhattacharyya T, Gale D, Dewire P, Totterman S, Gale ME, McLaughlin S, et al. The clinical importance of meniscal tears demonstrated by magnetic resonance imaging in osteoarthritis of the knee. J Bone Joint Surg Am 2003;85-A(1):4–9.

[74] Shelbourne KD, Wilckens JH. Intraarticular anterior cruciate ligament reconstruction in the symptomatic arthritic knee. Am J Sports Med 1993;21(5):685–8 [discussion 688–9].

[75] Noyes FR, Barber-Westin SD. Arthroscopic-assisted allograft anterior cruciate ligament reconstruction in patients with symptomatic arthrosis. Arthroscopy 1997;13(1):24–32.

[76] Shelbourne KD, Gray T. Results of anterior cruciate ligament reconstruction based on meniscus and articular cartilage status at the time of surgery. Five- to fifteen-year evaluations. Am J Sports Med 2000;28(4):446–52.

[77] Keene JS, Dyreby Jr JR. High tibial osteotomy in the treatment of osteoarthritis of the knee. The role of preoperative arthroscopy. J Bone Joint Surg Am 1983;65(1):36–42.

[78] Keene JS, Monson DK, Roberts JM, Dyreby Jr JR. Evaluation of patients for high tibial osteotomy. Clin Orthop 1989;243:157–65.
[79] Schultz W, Gobel D. Articular cartilage regeneration of the knee joint after proximal tibial valgus osteotomy: a prospective study of different intra- and extra-articular operative techniques. Knee Surg Sports Traumatol Arthrosc 1999;7(1):29–36.
[80] Williams III RJ, Wickiewicz TL, Warren RF. Management of unicompartmental arthritis in the anterior cruciate ligament-deficient knee. Am J Sports Med 2000;28(5):749–60.
[81] Akizuki S, Yasukawa Y, Takizawa T. Does arthroscopic abrasion arthroplasty promote cartilage regeneration in osteoarthritic knees with eburnation? A prospective study of high tibial osteotomy with abrasion arthroplasty versus high tibial osteotomy alone. Arthroscopy 1997; 13(1):9–17.

ELSEVIER
SAUNDERS

CLINICS
IN SPORTS
MEDICINE

Clin Sports Med 24 (2005) 153–161

Osteotomies around the Knee for the Young Athlete with Osteoarthritis

Michelle Wolcott, MD

Division of Sports Medicine, Department of Orthopaedic Surgery,
University of Colorado Health Sciences Center, 1745 S. High Street, Denver, CO 80210, USA

Jackson first described proximal tibial osteotomy in 1958 as a successful treatment for moderate to severe unicompartmental, degenerative arthritis of the knee associated with angular deformity [1]. Many studies have analyzed the results of this operation with respect to age, activity, gender, degree of arthritic changes, weight, previous injury treatment, and preoperative and postoperative angulation, in an effort to identify the risk factors for failure [2–5]. Evaluation of distal femoral osteotomy for valgus deformity has yielded similar results [6–10]. Findings indicate that factors predicting favorable outcomes include decreased relative weight, increased angle of correction, and lower overall level of disease. For the younger, active patient with angular deformity beyond the average range of physiologic variation, osteotomy remains the procedure of choice.

Pathophysiology

Osteoarthritis of the knee is generally considered to be a mechanical phenomenon. In the young adult, pathologic phenomenon such as meniscal injury, or meniscectomy, osteochondral injury, and ligamentous insufficiency can predispose an individual to develop osteoarthritis [11]. Changes in water content and decreased cartilage matrix synthesis lead to macroscopic fissuring and cartilage loss. Knee malalignment, whether induced by injury or underlying anatomic variability, has been shown to place abnormal stresses on the articular cartilage of an affected compartment and promote the development of these changes [12–15] (Fig. 1). The normal anatomic load-bearing axis of the knee ranges from

---

E-mail address: Michelle.Wolcott@uchsc.edu

0278-5919/05/$ – see front matter © 2004 Elsevier Inc. All rights reserved.
doi:10.1016/j.csm.2004.08.002   *sportsmed.theclinics.com*

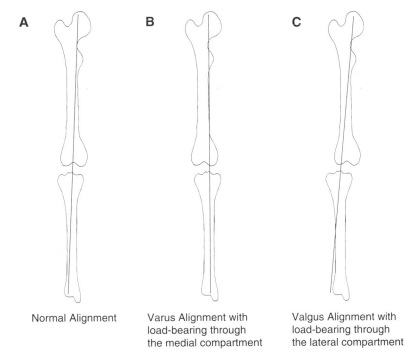

Fig. 1. Demonstration of various biomechanical axes. (*A*) Normal alignment. (*B*) Varus alignment with load bearing through the medial compartment. (*C*) Valgus alignment with load bearing through the lateral compartment.

5 to 7 degrees of valgus. The medial side of the knee bears 60% of the force transmitted through the joint, with 40% born laterally. Walking further increases the load by adding lateral thrust or an adduction moment varying somewhat by gait pattern [16]. Younger patients may be more prone to these changes resulting from injury in an isolated compartment, thus altering the biomechanical axis and accelerating this process. Total joint replacement remains a viable alternative for the older, less active patient, but long-term outcomes in the young adult have been less reliable and more complex. As a result, clinicians have recommended osteotomy as a means of altering malalignment to more evenly distribute these forces over both the medial and lateral compartment and delay or prevent degenerative changes in this population.

History

Age, weight, and activity level should be assessed in all patients as selection of appropriate surgical candidates may be influenced by these factors. Patients with unicompartmental arthritis generally complain of localized knee pain. A history of injury or previous surgery should be sought out. Pain may be vague in nature and related to repetitive, high-stress weight-bearing activites such as running or jumping. Seldom do symptoms occur with activities of daily living. Stiffness may or may not accompany pain, but more frequently occurs after prolonged immobilization. These patients often report significant relief with NSAIDS. More chronic symptoms may be more difficult to characterize, and may occur with lesser activities. Patients in this category will most often demonstrate more advanced disease. It is important to delineate the nature, location, and duration of pain symptoms. Advanced cartilage degeneration leads to advanced clinical symptoms, and should be correlated with radiographic findings.

Functional scoring may also be used to evaluate extent of disease. Commonly used rating scales for osteoarthritis include the WOMAC assessment, HSS knee score, and Knee Society knee score [17,18]. These evaluations have traditionally been used to evaluate older patients undergoing osteotomy or knee replacement surgery for pain associated with joint degeneration.

Physical examination

Examination of affected patients should include the following assessments: gait, stance, range of motion, localization of tenderness, ligamentous stability, neurologic evaluation, and lower extremity alignment. Classification as varus, valgus, or neutral alignment should be made. Unicompartmental osteoarthritis can be determined by localized joint line tenderness, crepitus, tenderness elicited with loading of the involved compartment, and joint space collapse. Ligamentous laxity may accompany joint space collapse, but may be related to loss of meniscal or cartilage height rather than true laxity. End point determination should be made to confirm integrity of the collateral ligaments.

Imaging studies

Preoperative radiologic assessment should be done with the patient upright in the weight-bearing, double-stance position. Full hip-to-ankle radiographs are obtained to determine the anatomic and mechanical axes of both the affected and unaffected extremity [16,19,20]. Weight-bearing AP, lateral, sunrise, and 40 degree flexion views are also obtained to assess joint space loss throughout a range of motion. Radiographic changes associated with osteoarthritis (loss of joint space, subchondral cysts, sclerosis, spurring) are noted. Occasionally, additional studies may be obtained to evaluate early changes. Bone scans may be useful in visualizing early unicompartmental disease. MRI may be used to evaluate cartilage or subchondral bone signal changes consistent with early osteoarthritis. Associated injuries such as mensical and ligamentous pathology can also be assessed.

Clinical approach

The recommended approach to young patients with clinically apparent unicompartmental osteoarthritis is to begin with conservative measures including activity modification when applicable, NSAIDS, and orthotic management. However, some amount of caution should be used in this approach. Oftentimes, surgical intervention is more successful when less disease progression is apparent [3,21]. Symptomatic disease may be more appropriately treated with a course of conservative therapy. Radiographic changes, however, should be used to alert the clinician to advancement of the disease. Indications for surgical intervention include young physiologic patient age, high demand activity level, malalignment beyond physiologic norms, and failure of conservative measures.

Preoperative planning

Surgery is considered in those patients who have failed conservative management, and in whom malalignment is radiographically confirmed. Proximal tibial osteotomies have been performed by a variety of methods that each employ some risk and benefit. The author's preferred method is a medial opening wedge tibial osteotomy using internal fixation and bone grafting. Advantages to this method include sparing of the proximal tibio-fibular joint and peroneal nerve, intraoperative adjustment if necessary, and avoidance of intraarticular pin placement (as with external fixation). Disadvantages include the need for bone graft and difficulty in correcting severe deformity. In the majority of young patients the amount of correction is mild, so that acute opening wedge osteotomy is acceptable. Similar risks and benefits apply to lateral opening wedge distal femoral osteotomy.

Using preoperative hip-to-ankle radiographs, the amount of correction can be determined by measuring the biomechanical axis of the affected extremity [22]. The width of the tibial plateau should be measured and marked at 62% from the medial or lateral side, depending on the direction of correction. This will be the location of the new weight-bearing axis of the extremity. A line is drawn from the center of the femoral head to this mark. In a similar fashion, a line is drawn from this mark to the center of the talus. The angle created by these two lines becomes the angle of correction.

Surgical technique for medial opening wedge tibial osteotomy

Surgery is performed under fluoroscopic guidance using a tourniquet. The patient is postioned supine, and normal surgical preparation is observed. An incision is made halfway between the tibial tubercle and the posteromedial border of the tibia. Dissection is carried down to the sartorius fascia. The fascia is incised in line with the fiber of the pes anserinus tendons, which are then retracted medially, exposing the superficial medial collateral ligament (MCL). A periosteal elevator is used to retract the MCL medially exposing the underlying tibial cortex. Anteriorly the patellar tendon is retracted laterally. The most superior fibers of the patellar tendon may be released to improve visualization of the osteoetomy site. A guide pin is placed using fluoroscopic guidance beginning 4 cm distal to the medial tibial plateau to a point approximately 1 cm distal to the lateral tibial plateau (at the level of the fibular head crossing proximal to the tibial tubercle). Orientation of this pin is marked to determine the angle of the osteotomy. An oscillating saw is placed below and parallel to the guide pin to begin the osteotomy taking care to cut only the medial and posteromedial cortex. Thin osteotomes are used to complete the osteotomy ending approximately 1 cm

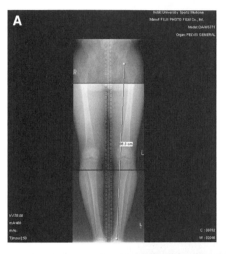

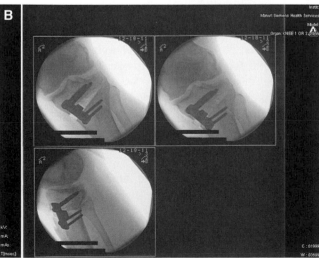

Fig. 2. A 36-year male with medial compartment pain and varus laxity. (*A*) Pre-op mechanical alignment. (*B*) Intraoperative fluoro. (*C*) Post-op mechanical axis. (*D*) Radiographic consolidation at 3 months post-op.

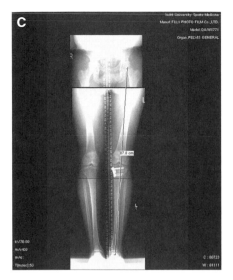
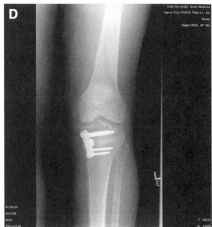

Fig. 2 (*continued*).

short of the lateral femoral cortex to maintain a lateral hinge. Larger osteotomes are then used to gradually open the osteotomy site. A calibrated osteotome is then used to open the osteotomy to the desired correction. A four-holed osteotomy plate (eg, Puddu, EBI) is then placed into the osteotomy site; 6.5 cancellous screws are placed through the proximal holes taking care not to violate the articular surface; 4.5 cortical screws are then used to fill the distal holes. Tricortical auto- or allograft is then placed into the defect. The wounds are then closed and the knee protected in a brace for 6 weeks. Weight-bearing should be delayed, but may be progressed to partial weight bearing during the intial 6 weeks, advancing to full weight bearing when radiographic consolidation is confirmed [23]. At this point, activity level can be increased to include strengthening and sport-specific drills. Return to sport can be determined based on specific sport criteria (Fig. 2).

Surgical technique for lateral opening wedge femoral osteotomy

Patient positioning and preparation are similar to that for proximal tibial osteotomy. An incision is made over the lateral aspect of the distal femur and carried down to the level of the iliotibial band. This is retracted anteriorly to expose the vastus lateralis. The posterior border of this muscle is identified and also retracted anteriorly to expose the lateral femoral cortex. Using the previously determined correction angle, an osteotomy is made in a similar fashion to that used for the proximal tibial osteotomy. An opening wedge is created to realign the mechanical axis and fixation is accomplished as above. Postoperative regimen remains the same.

Clinical results

Results of proximal tibial osteotomy have been uniformly good when the proper correction is maintained in the appropriate patient and no complications have ensued. Unlike other procedures for osteoarthritis, proximal tibial osteotomy allows the patient significant, if not unlimited, activity. Results in different populations of patients have been variable. Initial studies assessing results of proximal tibial osteotomies have shown deterioration of results beyond 10 years [4,21]. More recent studies, however, have shown that various risk factors may play a role in maintaining success rates and improvement of knee scores over time. Risk factors that seem to lead to unfavorable outcomes include increased relative body weight, progression of disease before intervention, and under- or overcorrection of alignment [2–4,24,25]. No study has been able to determine a significant relationship between outcome and patient age. Some speculation asserts that improved results can be indirectly attributed to decreased severity of disease and increased activity level in the younger patient population.

Complications

The observed complication rate for proximal tibial osteotomy is highly variable, and falls into two categories: complications related to the surgical procedure, and failure of the procedure. Reported surgical complication rates are low and include nonunion of osteotomy, transient peroneal nerve palsy (lateral closing wedge osteotomies), pin tract infection, and DVTs. Long-term post surgical results, however, are less favorable. Various failure rates in pain relief and progression to total joint replacement are more closely correlated with undercorrection of the mechanical axis [2–4,21,24,25]. Less common failures are reported with overcorrection [2]. There have been no well-designed long-term studies in younger patients to determine accurate failure rates, but early evidence suggests increasing long-term benefit with proper correction of malalignment in patients with early degenerative changes [23,24].

Summary

Younger patients sustaining injury to articular surfaces are at increased risk of degenerative changes. Underlying or resultant malalignment can compound this problem, leading to increased unicompartmental contact pressures and cartilage degeneration. Surgical options have become increasingly popular, as recent studies have suggested that early surgical intervention leads to better long-term results. Total joint replacement has been shown to improve functional outcome scores in the older and less active patient; however, the younger, more active patient presents a more difficult problem. Correction of malalignment in isolated unicompartmental disease has shown encouraging results. More long-term studies are needed to determine the functional results of this procedure in this evolving patient population.

References

[1] Jackson JP, Waugh W, Green JP. High tibial osteotomy for osteoarthritis of the knee. J Bone Joint Surg 1969;51B:88–94.

[2] Matthews LS, Goldstein SA, Malvitz TA, Katz BP, Kaufer H. Proximal tibial osteotomy: factors that influence the duration of satisfactory function. Clin Orthop 1988;229:193–200.

[3] Holden DL, James SL, Larson RL, Slocum DB. Proximal tibial osteotomy in patients who are fifty years old or less: a long-term follow up study. J Bone Joint Surg 1988;70A:977–82.

[4] Coventry MB, Ilstrup DM, Wallrichs SL. Proximal tibial osteotomy. A critical long-term study. J Bone Joint Surg 1993;75A:196–201.

[5] Aglietti P, Rinonapoli E, Stringa G, Taviani A. Tibial osteotomy for the varus osteoarthritic knee. Clin Orthop 1983;176:239.

[6] Edgerton B, Mariani E, Morrey B. Distal femoral varus osteotomy for painful genu valgum. A five-to-11 year follow-up study. Clin Orthop 1993;288:263–9.

[7] Maquet P. The treatment of choice in osteoarthritis of the knee. Clin Orthop 1985;192:108–12.

[8] McDermott A, Finklestein J, Farine I, Boynton EL, MacIntosh DL, Gross A. Distal femoral varus osteotomy for valgus deformity of the knee. J Bone Joint Surg 1988;70:110–6.

[9] Phillips M, Krackow K. High tibial osteotomy and distal femoral osteotomy for valgus or varus deformity around the knee. Instr Course Lect 1998;47:429–35.

[10] Aglietti P, Menchetti P. Distal femoral varus osteotomy in the valgus osteoarthritic knee. Am J Knee Surg 2000;13:89–95.

[11] Allen PR, Denham RA, Swan AV. Late degenerative changes after meniscectomy. Factors affecting knee after operation. J Bone Joint Surg 1984;66B:666–71.

[12] Phillips MJ, Krackow KA. High tibial osteotomy and distal femoral osteotomy for valgus and varus deformity around the knee. Instr Course Lect 1998;47:429–36.

[13] Reimann I. Experimental osteoarthritis of the knee in rabbits induced by alteration of the load-bearing. Acta Orthop Scand 1973;44:496–504.

[14] Tetsworth K, Paley D. Malalignment and degenerative arthropathy. Orthop Clin North Am 1994;25:367–77.

[15] Wu DD, Burr DB, Boyd RB, Radin EL. Bone and cartilage changes following experimental varus or valgu tibial angulation. J Orthop Res 1990;8:572–85.

[16] Coventry M. Upper tibial osteotomy for osteoarthritis. J Bone Joint Surg 1985;67A:1136–40.

[17] Insall JN, Dorr LD, Scott RD, Scott WN. Rationale of the Knee Society clinical rating system. Clin Orthop 1989;248:13–4.

[18] Roos EM, Roos HP, Lohmander LS. WOMAC Osteoarthritis Index – additional dimensions for use in subjects with post-traumatic osteoarthritis of the knee. Osteoarthritis Cartilage 1999; 7:216–21.

[19] Fujisawa Y, Masuhara K, Shiomi S. The effect of high tibial osteotomy on osteoarthritis of the knee: an arthroscopic study of 54 knee joints. Orthop Clin North Am 1979;10:585–608.

[20] Insall JN, Joseph DM, Msika C. High tibial osteotomy for varus gonarthrosis. A long-term follow-up study. J Bone Joint Surg 1984;66A:1040–8.

[21] Rudan JF, Simurda MA. Valgus high tibial osteotomy: a long-term follow-up study. Clin Orthop 1991;268:157–60.

[22] Dugdale TW, Noyes FR, Styer D. Preoperative planning for high tibial osteotomy. The effect of lateral tibiofemoral separation and tibiofemoral length. Clin Orthop 1992;274:248–64.

[23] Amendola A, Mrkonjic L, Clatworthy M, Kirkley A. Opening wedge high tibial osteotomy using a Puddu distraction plate: focus on technique, early results and complications. Presented

at the International Society of Arthroscopy, Knee Surgery and Orthopaedic Sports Medicine, Washington (DC): 1999.

[24] Yasuda K, Majima T, Tsuchida T, Kaneda K. A ten to 15-year follow up observation of high tibial osteotomy in medial compartment osteoarthritis. Clin Orthop 1992;282:186–95.

[25] Ivarsson I, Myrnerts R, Gilquist J. High tibial osteotomy for medial osteoarthritis of the knee: a 5 to 7 and an 11 to 13 year follow-up. J Bone Joint Surg 1990;72B:238–44.

ELSEVIER
SAUNDERS

Clin Sports Med 24 (2005) 163–174

CLINICS
IN SPORTS
MEDICINE

Surgical Management of Cartilage Defects in Athletes

Paul K. Ritchie, MD, MS, Eric C. McCarty, MD*

*University of Colorado School of Medicine, Department of Orthopaedics,
CU Sports Medicine and Shoulder Surgery, 311 Mapleton Avenue, Boulder, CO 80304, USA*

The synovial joints provide a unique environment in which to carry out their critical mechanical function. The complex architecture of the articular cartilage normally provides painless motion throughout a variety of activities. Fluids secreted by cells in the superficial layers of the articular cartilage as well as in the synovium provide an almost frictionless articulation [1]. The synovium also helps to maintain the aseptic environment found within the joint. The cartilage and fluid provide critical protection to the underlying bone. If any of these structures are damage, or lose their efficiency, the ensuing cascade of damage inflicted on the joint can lead to catastrophic failure [2].

The articular cartilage is often innocently under constant attack in our ever-ncreasingly active population. This activity is amplified in athletes, which often places increased demands on the critical functions of the articular cartilage and joints. The repetitive nature of individual competition and training can often lead to microinjury and damage to many of the specialized cells and scaffolding of the extracellular matrix of articular cartilage. Increased weight and muscle strength directed to the bones, coupled with frequent high-energy collisions and torsional movements by the athlete often leads to increased stresses transmitted directly to the cartilage complex, potentially speeding its destruction. Injury to the cartilage often leads to shearing, compression, or avulsion of articular cartilage in the athlete [3].

The orthopedist will frequently encounter chondral or osteochondral injuries while caring for active patients, and it behooves the surgeon to be prepared to treat these injuries. In a review of 31,516 knee arthroscopies performed over a

* Corresponding author.
E-mail address: Eric.mccarty@uchsc.edu (E.C. McCarty).

0278-5919/05/$ – see front matter © 2004 Elsevier Inc. All rights reserved.
doi:10.1016/j.csm.2004.08.013
sportsmed.theclinics.com

4.5-year period, Curl et al documented 53,569 hyaline cartilaginous lesions in 19,827 (63%) of the study patients. Interestingly, 5% of all arthroscopies involved patients under the age of 40 who demonstrated grade IV lesions [4]. The constellation of articular cartilage damage ranges from a simple contusion to fracture and fissuring through the articular cartilage and subchondral bone. As pointed out by Farmer et al, these injuries have often gone undiagnosed in the past [5], and any delay in diagnosis and treatment can further exacerbate the injury. Therefore, a high index of suspicion for a potential articular cartilaginous injury must be maintained while examining and evaluating an active patient with joint pain. A careful physical exam as well as appropriate imaging modalities is critical to make the appropriate diagnosis.

Surgical management

Intuitively, one understands that a lesion of any size in the smooth surface of the articular cartilage can lead to perturbations in the normal mechanical functioning of the cartilage cap. Increased pressures are concentrated on the cartilage surrounding the lesion, normal matrix interactions become interrupted, and ultimately, an increase in the rate of cartilage deterioration and osteoarthritis can ensue. Once the determination has been made of articular cartilage damage, and the lesion appropriately classified, the surgeon contemplates the type of cartilage repair that will be attempted [6]. As Browne et al has pointed out; the various treatment options can be stratified into the two general categories of restorative or reparative. The goal of a restorative surgical technique is a complete reconstruction of the microarchitecture, physiology, and biomechanics of the articular cartilage, thus providing relief of symptoms. A reparative technique relies on the restoration of differing aspects of articular cartilage function and form without completely restoring all architectural and physiologic properties [7]. The various treatment options include excision with irrigation, debridement, and abrasion chondroplasty, bone marrow stimulation techniques (microfracture), radiofrequency ablation/debridement, periosteal grafting, autologous chondrocyte transplantation, and autogenous osteochondral grafting (mosaicplasty) or allografting (fresh frozen allografts).

Irrigation, debridement, abrasion chondroplasty

Several studies have noted that patients that undergo arthroscopic lavage of an injured joint demonstrate an improvement in symptoms [8,9]. It must be noted that a few studies have reported an inherent placebo effect by the procedure of arthroscopic lavage when used in the treatment of osteoarthritis [10,11]. These studies should not be taken to infer that arthroscopic lavage in an acutely injured joint relies on a similar placebo effect as may be seen in the chronic process of degenerative osteoarthritis. These two pathologies should be considered as completely separate entities, and receive different treatment algorithms. In a joint with an articular cartilage defect, arthroscopic lavage helps to remove the various inflammatory mediators, and metalloproteases present in the joint fluid.

The addition of debridement with lavage can further improve symptoms by allowing the removal of loose bodies, free flaps, or any loose cartilage in the lesion. Abrasion chondroplasty attempts to create a full-thickness lesion down into the subchondral bone at the site of injury. This resulting completed lesion is hoped to then stimulate repair through infiltration of cells within the joint space, ultimately resulting in the formation of reparative tissue of fibrocartilage to fill the void [12,13]. Problems with this technique include the destruction of much of the subchondral plate, difficulty in controlling the depth of penetration, and the overgrowth of fibrocartilage covering an uneven bone bed. These modalities should not be applied as the sole treatment, as they often do not appropriately address the resulting articular surface defect. As previously discussed, a defect in the articular surface can lead to further lesion progression and joint carti-lage degeneration.

Marrow stimulation techniques (microfracture)

This technique relies on the infiltration of pleuripotent mesenchymal stem cells to provide a type of restorative cartilage growth into a cartilage defect. The technique has been used in the various patient groups including most significantly, the highly trained and conditioned athletic population. The technique as described by Steadman et al involves the use of specially designed sharp awls used arthroscopically to make multiple perforations, or microfractures, into the subchondral bone in a controlled fashion [14]. Success of the technique relies on maintenance of an intact subchondral plate. Awls are used in place of drilling or abrasion to provide a sharp puncture in the subchondral bone without inducing thermal injury and necrosis. These perforations are placed as closed to one another without causing interval plate fracture, or violation into another perforation. These small perforations then allow the egress of bone marrow elements, including growth factors, mesenchymal pleuripotent stem cells, and various humeral stimulating factors. This pro-genesis milieu then forms the important "super clot" that provides nature's cradle of the appropriately enriched environment for the ensuing growth of reparative tissue. The technique can be used to treat lesions on all the articular surfaces of the knee including the patella and trochlear groove [15].

The rehabilitation program used in conjunction with the technique is critical for its success [16]. The rehab protocol requires strict nonweight bearing for the first 8 weeks. Continuous passive motion is also used during these 8 weeks for a minimum of 6 to 8 hours per day. It is felt that this controlled motion, without the compression of weight bearing, allows the nescient stem cells in the super clot, with their accompanying growth factors, to differentiate and proliferated into an appropriate "articular cartilage-like" cell line to fill the defect [14,15]. The technique has demonstrated ability to improve function and symptoms in various patients including professional athletes [17,18]. In a study of patients age 13 to 45, who presented with full-thickness traumatic defects without meniscus or ligamentous pathology, Steadman demonstrated statistically significant improvement in function and pain when compared with their pretreatment condition. At 7 years, 80% of the patients considered themselves improved in pain [18]. When choosing this treatment modality, it is important to remember that the cartilage that forms consists predominately of fibrocartilage. The mechanical characteristics of fibrocartilage differ from normal hyaline articular cartilage in its ability to withstand compressive and sheering forces. There are no large, randomized, or controlled studies involving this technique, and future study will be helpful in defining the appropriate parameters for its use.

Radiofrequency ablation/debridement

This treatment modality is based on the observations that cartilage defects that do not penetrate completely through the articular surface down to the subchondral bone show little ability to repair itself without intervention. These lesions often continue to propagate down to the subchondral bone through delamination, fragmentation, and fibrillation. Rather than use knives, biters, curettes, or rotary shavers to remove loose and irregular articular cartilage, several authors have employed the use of radiofrequency generated energy for arthroscopic soft tissue ablation, shrinkage of fibrillations, and smoothing of irregularities [19,20]. Great care and skill must be exercised when using this technique. Resent studies have demonstrated that the technique is both energy and time dependent. A very small increase in either the energy delivered, or the time the energy is delivered to the articular surface increases the depth and extent of cellular death [21]. Other studies have shown that both Monopolar and Bipolar radiofrequency energy delivered to the articular cartilage can cause significant cell death to various depths including down to the subchondral bone [22,23]. Studies have shown clinical improvement in knees treated with bipolar radiofrequency energy versus those treated with mechanical debridement, with less cartilage death when bipolar energy is used [24,25]. In light of the questions and conflicts posed by these studies, the long-term effects of this treatment modality needs further scrutiny to determine the appropriate indications and usage of this technology.

Periosteal grafting

This technique uses transplantation of the periosteum with its rich cellular components into a cartilaginous defect. These cells in the periosteal matrix include pleuripotent-undifferentiated cells that have the potential to form cartilage. When placed in the appropriate avascular environment with the appropriate mechanical stimulus, these cells grow and developed into various forms of cartilage. O'Driscoll has pointed out the numerous technical considerations when using this technique. The graft must be carefully harvested, and fixed into the defect with the cambium layer facing into the joint. Postoperative treatment of continuous passive motion is important to stimulate the appropriate cartilage formation [26]. There are relatively few human studies discussing results of this technique in humans, and further research in conjunction with tissue engineering principles will provide further cartilage repair and restoration options.

Autologous chondrocyte implantation

The treatment of cartilage defects in the knee with the transplantation of autologous chondrocytes was first reported in a 1994 study by Brittberg et al [27]. This technique involves the harvesting of cartilage cells from an uninvolved area of the joint in an initial arthroscopic procedure. The cells are then grown and multiplied in culture medium in the laboratory for several weeks multiplying the cells 10- to 20-fold. These cultured cells are then reimplanted into the cartilage defect underneath a periosteal flap that has been harvested, transplanted from proximal bone, and sown into place covering the defect during a second open procedure. Postoperative motion allows the cells to grow a "hyaline-like" and fibrocartilaginous articular cartilage to fill the defect.

Several authors have reported promising results using autologous chondrocyte implantation (ACI) techniques. Minas reported on a prospective cohort evaluation of 169 patients ranging in age from 13 to 58 years old. The patients were stratified into the categories of simple, complex, and salvage based on the size and number of lesions. Numerous patient assessment instruments were used to evaluate the outcome. Patient satisfaction at 24 months was 60% for simple, 70% for complex, and 90% for salvage categories. Interestingly, there were only 22 (13%) failures, defined as no clinical improvement or graft failure [28]. Brittberg et al discussed the follow-up of 244 consecutive patients stratified into various subgroups based on location, number, and size of lesions from 2 to 10 years. This study demonstrates that ACI gave a high percentage of good to excellent results (84–90%) in patients with different types of single femoral condyle lesions. Patients with other types of lesions such as the patella and trochlea have demonstrated lower degrees of success (74%) [29,30]. Micheli et al reported on the use of ACI in the pediatric population of ages 10 to 17 years old with a mean age of 15 years of age. This study involved 32 patients with follow-up for at least 2 years. In this small group of juvenile patients there was significant improvement in baseline, pain, and swelling scores [31].

The rehabilitation process after ACI includes continuous passive motion and a program of gradually increasing the patients weight-bearing status. Protection of the grafted material is crucial during the initial few weeks. All twisting, rotational, and shearing forces must be avoided. Protocols gradually progress the patient to rigorous activity by 12 to 15 months.

In this era of cost containment the significant expense of culturing the chondrocytes can present a prohibitive barrier to widespread implementation of this technique. The procedure requires careful attention to details, and meticulous preparation of the lesion before grafting. Results are best if the subchondral bone remains intact. Care must be taken to minimize bleeding in the lesion to decrease the infiltration of fibrocytes and the ensuing fibrocartilage growth in the transplanted cells and the resulting tissue. The procedure is limited by the ability of the transplanted cells to grow, proliferate, differentiate, and form and maintain attachment at the implantation site. There is great need to find materials and biologic scaffolds that can maintain these grafted cells in the defect, as well as enhance their ability to proliferate and differentiate. New areas of study include anatomically shaped osteochondral constructs, as well as investigation and development of the various cytokines and other intra- and extracellular signaling chemicals that influence and regulate articular cartilage cell growth [32].

Osteochondral autografts (oats, mosaicplasty)

The successful treatment of articular cartilage lesions using the transplantation of one or more autologous osteochondral plugs (mosaicplasty) has been demonstrated by several authors [33,34]. This technique involves removing small osteochondral plugs from the periphery of the patellofemoral joint, or along the margins of the intercondylar notch, and transplanting them into areas of articular cartilage defect in the weight bearing areas of the joint. This construct allows the maintenance of the articular cartilage/subchondral bone interface. When performed properly, the plug, or plugs, allows the restoration of the normal contact pressures of the articular surface, relieves pressure points, and helps normalize the joint back to a normal, smooth gliding surface.

Several studies have shown the clinical utility with positive results using the osteochondral autograft technique [35]. In a study by Hangody et al, 831 mosaicplasty procedures were performed. Clinical scores, imaging techniques, second-look arthroscopies, histologic examination of biopsy samples, and cartilage stiffness measurements were used to evaluate the clinical outcomes and quality of the transplanted cartilage. In this study, 92% of femoral condylar implantations, 87% of tibial resurfacing mosaicplasties, 79% of treated patellar or trochlear lesions, and 94% of talar lesions showed good to excellent results. Of note, 3% of the study patients showed long-term donor site disturbances. In 83 of the patients a second-look arthroscopy was performed for various reasons. In 69 of the 83 patients there was noted congruent gliding surfaces, histologically proven survival of the transplanted hyaline cartilage, and fibrocartilage covering of the donor sites [36,37].

The method has proven to be a valid option in the treatment of full-thickness lesions. It is technically demanding, and requires that the plugs be placed snuggly in a press-fit fashion, level with the surrounding cartilage, and at a true perpendicular angle to the articular surface restoring the normal curvature of the articular surface. There is the potential for donor-site morbidity, and it can be extremely difficult to restore the articular surface contour when reconstructing larger defects using multiple plugs. Thus, in the hands of most surgeons, the method is limited to defects of smaller sizes.

Osteochondral allografts

Osteochondral allografts are useful in treating cartilage injuries that are of larger size, or where there has been more extensive disruption of the subchondral bone. It is often used as a salvage procedure when other therapies have been attempted and failed, and can be useful after high-energy trauma and fractures. Several biologic factors of osteochondral grafts are responsible for their success in cartilage transplantation. The grafts are composite grafts of living chondrocytes and bone as an attachment vehicle. The chondrocytes are immunoprivileged and survive transplantation and support the mature hyaline matrix. The allograft bone is slowly replaced by host bone through the process of creeping substitution.

Aubin et al describes the long-term results of using fresh femoral osteochondral allografts to treat traumatic knee defects. In this report of 72 patients, 60 patients were available for follow-up (mean of 10 years). Survivorship analysis showed 85% graft survival at 10 years, and 74% survival at 15 years. Patients with surviving grafts had good function, and a mean Hospital for Special Surgery score of 83 points at 10 years follow-up [38]. In a review of 126 procedures on 123 knees, Gross demonstrated good or excellent results in 95% of patients at 5 years, 71% at 10 years, and 66% at 20 years [39].

The technical constraints of surgical implantation of fresh osteochondral allografts are extremely demanding. The graft must be properly matched to the site of implantation and fitted properly. Fresh allografts provide the greatest likelihood of chondrocyte survivability, but also increase the risk of transmissible diseases and infections. The chondrocytes in the graft demonstrate less viability the longer the graft is stored; basically, the viability decreases significantly after 28 days. Therefore, the patient, and surgeon must be ready on short notice when the appropriate donor graft becomes available for rapid placement of the allograft. As pointed out by Gross, the best indications for fresh osteochondral allografts may be in a large posttraumatic lesion, or in a larger osteochondritis dissecans defect [39].

Comparative studies

There has been a pronounced dearth of randomized controlled comparative studies regarding the treatment of articular cartilage defects in the orthopaedic literature. Many of the recently developed treatment options and techniques are relatively new with few published studies. There are also few studies with sufficient numbers of patients to allow comparisons of the various treatments, and draw conclusions about the significance of observed differences in outcomes. As these studies emerge, they warrant careful scrutiny.

Two prospective randomized studies comparing osteochondral transplantation versus ACI achieved opposite conclusions. A study by Horas et al demonstrated that both treatments result in a decrease in symptoms. The improvement provided by the ACI lagged behind that provided by the mosaicplasty. Also, they noted that histologically, the defects treated with ACI were primarily filled with fibrocartilage, whereas the mosaicplasty transplants retained their hyaline character [40]. A study by Bentley et al, using various outcome measurements, determined that 88% of patients that had ACI treatment demonstrated good or excellent results, versus 69% of the patients treated with mosaicplasty. Arthroscopy at 1 year demonstrated excellent or good repairs in 82% after ACI, and in 34% after mosaicplasty. All five of the patellar mosaicplasties in the study failed. They concluded that in this study ACI demonstrated significant superiority versus mosaicplasty. It is interesting to note the different conclusion by the two studies. Several factors will lead to these types of differences such as variations in lesion size and location, difference in the functional outcome measurement tools used, differences in rehabilitation protocols, and differences in patients' age, size, and expectations, and compliance. Each study should be reviewed on its individual merits.

Several recent studies have compared ACI versus the microfracture technique. Coleman et al presented a study providing clinical and MR comparison of ACI versus microfracture [41]. A physical examination and the modified Cincinnati Knee Questionnaire were used to determine clinical outcome. The Cincinnati scores improved an average of 22% for the ACI treatment group, and 42% for the microfracture treated group. The average MR score for the ACI group was 66%, versus 44% for the microfracture group. A score of 100% represents normal articular cartilage. There was a greater clinical improvement in the group treated with the microfracture technique compared with the patient receiving ACI. This clinical improvement did not correlate with MR findings. A study comparing ACI to microfracture by Anderson et al demonstrated a significantly greater improvement from baseline in the overall condition score of the ACI versus microfracture patients [42].

A recent comparison study by Knutsen et al showed no difference in the patient outcomes between the two methods of treatment. The International Cartilage Repair Society, Lysholm, SF-36, and Tegner forms were use to collect data. Independent observers performed the follow-up examinations, and 84% of the study population underwent biopsy of the treatment area. The histologic evaluation of repair tissues showed no macroscopic or significant histologic differences between the two groups. The SF-36 physical component score noted a significantly better improvement in the microfracture group than that in the ACI group at 2 years. Otherwise, there was no significant difference in the two methods, and both methods had acceptable short-term results [43]. As comparative studies continue to emerge, they will be helpful to continually redefine the clinical setting in which each technique will be most useful. As previously stated, their usefulness will increase as the numerous variables are held as constant as possible across the study patients.

Summary

There has been tremendous discussion attempting to determine what constitutes the appropriate treatment for this challenging clinical problem. Several authors have presented various opinions for pleasantly plausible repair algorithms [5,7,44–47]. Rather than recapitulate their work, it is helpful to consider restorative and reparative options in general terms of their possible judicious applications.

Any potential procedure must be carefully analyzed for appropriateness, and potential to repair the cartilage defect, or restore the articular surface. The size, depth, and location of the articular lesion must first be considered. Several factors described by Alleyne et al such as advanced age, workers compensation involvement, obesity, and large lesions involving a significant percentage of the articular surface represent negative prognosticators [47]. Tantamount for the success of any cartilage restorative procedure, any issues of malalignment must be addressed before, or in conjunction with, the restoration of the articular surface. Continued nonphysiologic pressures on a lesion due to malalignment will doom any endeavor to repair the articular cartilage. A careful discussion must be undertaken with the patient to describe and discuss possible treatment options, procedure morbidity associated with each treatment option (ie, pain, stiffness, cosmesis, blood loss, or lost time from work or sport), as well as determine the patients expectations from the surgical management in the treatment of the articular cartilage damage [47,48].

Ultimately, it behooves the surgeon to consider all therapeutic options, as the best success will be obtained when a treatment is selected and individualized according to the extent and type of lesion, as well as the patients needs, expectations, and ability and willingness to comply with rehabilitation protocols. As a surgeon, the restoration of the articular surface offers a tremendous opportunity to provide a substantial impact on a patient's well-being in a vastly positive fashion. As we often receive daily instructions, and are tutored by our ministrations and observations of our patients, we quickly learn that damage to the articular cartilage is often the cause of an athlete's inability to compete at a high level, and can often lead to career demise and early retirement. It is most imperative that we continue to expand our knowledge and abilities, as well as develop improved techniques to repair and restore this astoundingly resilient yet delicate covering of the articular surface of the joints.

References

[1] Buckwalter JA, Mankin HJ. Articular cartilage I: tissue design and chondrocyte–matrix interactions. J Bone Joint Surg 1997;79A(4):600–11.

[2] Buckwalter JA, Mankin HJ. Articular cartilage II: degeneration and osteoarthrosis, repair, regeneration and transplantation. J Bone Joint Surg 1997;79A(4):612–32.

[3] Mow VC, Zhu W, Ratcliffe A. Basic orthopaedic biomechanics. In: Mow VC, Zhu W, editors. Structure and function of articular cartilage and meniscus. New York: Raven Press; 1991. p. 1–453.

[4] Curl WW, Krome J, Gordon ES, Rushing J, Smith BP, Poehling GG. Cartilage injuries: a review of 31,516 knee arthroscopies. Arthroscopy 1997;13(4):456–60.

[5] Farmer JM, Martin DF, Boles CA, Curl WW. Chondral and osteochondral injuries. Clin Sports Med 2001;20(2):299–319.

[6] Poole AR. What type of cartilage repair are we attempting to attain? J Bone Joint Surg Am 2003;85-A(Suppl 2):40–4.

[7] Browne JE, Branch TP. Surgical alternatives for treatment of articular cartilage lesions. J Am Acad Orthop Surg 2000;8:180–9.

[8] Bauer M, Jackson RW. Chondral lesions of the femoral condyles: a system of arthroscopic classification. Arthroscopy 1988;4:97–102.

[9] McGinty J, editor. Operative arthroscopy. 2nd edition. Philadelphia: Lippincott Williams and Wilkins; 1994.

[10] Moseley JB, Wray NP, Kuykendall D, Willis K, Landon G. Arthroscopic treatment of osteoarthritis of the knee: a prospective, randomized, placebo-controlled trial. Results of a pilot study. Am J Sports Med 1996;24:28–34.

[11] Moseley JB, O'Malley K, Petersen NJ, Menke TJ, Brody BA, Kuykendall DH, et al. A controlled trial or arthroscopic surgery for osteoarthritis of the knee. N Engl J Med 2002;347(2): 81–8.

[12] Johnson L. Arthroscopic abrasion arthroplasty: historical and pathological perspective: present status. Arthroscopy 1986;2:54–69.

[13] Johnson LL. Arthroscopic abrasion arthroplasty. In: McGinty JB, Caspari RB, Jackson RW, Peohling GG, editors. Operative arthrscopy. 2nd edition. Philadelphia: Lippincott-Raven; 1996. p. 427–46.

[14] Steadman JR, Rodkey WG, Rodrigo JJ. Microfracture: surgical technique and rehabilitation to treat chondral defects. Clin Orthop 2001;391S:S362–9.

[15] Sledge SL. Microfracture techniques in the treatment of osteochondral injuries. Clin Sports Med 2001;20(2):365–77.

[16] Irrgang JJ, Pezzullo D. Rehabilitation following surgical prodedures to address articular cartilage lesions of the knee. J Orthop Sports Phys Ther 1998;28:232–40.

[17] Blevins FT, Steadman JR, Rodrigo JJ, Silliman J. Treatment of articular cartilage defects in athletes: an analysis of functional outcome and lesion appearance. Orthopedics 1998;21:761–8.

[18] Steadman JR, Briggs KK, Rodrigo JJ, Kocher MS, Gill TJ, Rodkey WG. Outcomes of microfracture for traumatic chondral defects of the knee: average 11-year follow-up. Arthroscopy 2003;19(5):477–84.

[19] Tasto JP, Ash SA. Current uses of radiofrequency in arthroscopic knee surgery. J Knee Surg 1999;12(3):186–91.

[20] Kaplan L, Uribe JW, Sasken H, Markarian G. The acute effects of radiofrequency energy in articular cartilage: an in vitro study. Arthroscopy 2000;16(1):2–5.

[21] Vangsness CT, Caffey S, Moore B, Hedman T. Effects of radiofrequency energy on human articular cartilage: an analysis of five systems. Presented at Annual Meeting of the American Academy of Orthopaedic Surgeons, Dallas (TX), February 13–17, 2002.

[22] Lu Y, Edwards RB, Cole BJ, Markel MD. Thermal chondroplasty with radiofrequency energy: an in vitro comparison of bipolar and monopolar radiofrequency devices. Am J Sports Med 2001;29(1):42–9.

[23] Lu Y, Hayashi D, Hecht P, Fanton GS, Thabit G, Cooley AJ, et al. The effect of monopolar radiofrequency energy on partial-thickness defects of articular cartilage. Arthroscopy 2000; 16(5):527–36.

[24] Gundel J, Saskin H, Popovitz L, Boldstein J, Yetkinler D, Frenkel S, et al. The effect of bipolar radiofrequency energy on partial-thickness chondral defects in a sheep model. Presented at 20th Annual Meeting of the Arthroscopy Association of North America, Seattle (WA), April 19–22, 2001.

[25] Owens BD, Stickles BJ, Balikian P, Busconi BD. Prospective analysis of radiofrequency versus mechanical debridement of isolated patellar chondral lesions. Presented at 20th Annual Meeting of the Arthroscopy Association of North Americam, Seattle (WA), April 19–22, 2001.

[26] O'Driscoll SW. Technical considerations in periosteal grafting for osteochondral injuries. Clin Sports Med 2001;20(2):379–402.

[27] Brittberg M, Lindahl A, Nilsson A, Ohlsson C, Isaksson O, Peterson L. Treatment of deep cartilage defects in the knee with autologous chondrocyte transplantation. N Engl J Med 1994; 331:889–95.

[28] Minas T. Autologous chondrocyte implantation for focal chondral defects of the knee. Clin Orthop 2001;391S:S349–61.

[29] Brittberg M, Tallheden T, Sjogren-Jansson E, Lindahl A, Peterson L. Autologous chondrocytes used for articular cartilage repair. Clin Orthop 2001;391S:S337–48.

[30] Brittberg M, Peterson L, Sjogren-Jansson E, Tallheden T, Lindah A. Articular cartilage engineering with autologous chondrocyte transplantation. J Bone Joint Surg 2003;85A(Suppl 3): 109–15.

[31] Micheli LJ, Moseley B, Anderson AF, Browne JE, Erggelet C, Arciero RA, et al. Articular cartilage defects in young patients: treatment with autologous chondrocyte implantation. Presented at 71st Annual Meeting of the American Academy of Orthopaedic Surgeons, San Francisco (CA), March 10–14, 2004.

[32] Hung CT, Lima EG, Mauck RL, Taki E, LeRoux MA, Lu HH, et al. Anatomically shaped osteochondral constructs for articular cartilage repair. J Biomech 2003;36(12):1853–64.

[33] Hangody L, Kish G, Karpati Z, Udvarhelyi I, Szigeti I, Bely M. Mosaicplasty for the treatment of articular cartilage defects: application in clinical practice. Orthopedics 1998;21:751–6.

[34] Kish G, Modis L, Hangody L. Osteochondral mosaicplasty for the treatment of focal chondral and osteochondral lesions of the knee and talus in the athlete: rationale, indications, techniques, and results. Clin Sports Med 1999;18:45–66.

[35] Jakob RP, Franz T, Gautier E, Mainil-Varlet P. Autologous osteochondral grafting in the knee: indication, results, and reflections. Clin Orthop 2002;401:170–84.

[36] Hangody L, Fules P. Autologous osteochondral Mosaicplasty for the treatment of full-thickness defects of weight-bearing joints: ten years of experimantal and clinical experience. J Bone Joint Surg 2003;85A(Suppl 2):25–32.

[37] Hangody L, Feczko P, Bartha L, Bodo G, Kish G. Mosaicplasty for the treatment of articular defects of the knee and ankle. Clin Orthop 2001;391S:S328–36.

[38] Aubin PP, Cheah HK, Davis AM, Gross AE. Long-term followup of fresh femoral osteochondral allografts for posttaumatic knee defects. Clin Orthop 2001;391S:S318–27.

[39] Gross AE. Fresh osteochondral allografts for post-traumatic knee defects: surgical technique. Operat Tech Orthop 1997;7:334–9.

[40] Hoaras U, Pelinkovic D, Herr G, Aigner T, Schnettler R. Autologous chondrocyte implantation and osteochondral cylinder transplantation in cartilage repair of the knee joint. A prospective, comparative trial. J Bone Joint Surg Am 2003;85A(2):185–92.

[41] Coleman SH, Malizia R, Potter H, MacGillivray JD, Warren RF. Treatment of isolated articular cartilage lesions of the medial femoral condyle—a clinical and MR comparison of autologous chondrocyte implantation vs microfracture. Presented at the Annual Meeting of the American Academy of Orthopaedic Surgeons, Dallas (TX), February 13–17, 2002.

[42] Anderson AF, Fu FH, Mandelbaum B, Browne JE, Moseley B, Erggelet C, et al. A controlled study of autologous chondrocyte implantation versus microfracture for articular cartilage lesions

of the femur. Presented at the 70th Annual Meeting of the American Academy of Orthopaedic Surgeons, New Orleans (LA), February 5–9, 2003.

[43] Knutsen G, Engebntsen L, Ludvigsen TC, Drogset JO, Grontuedt T, Solheim E, et al. Autologous chondrocyte implantation compared with microfracture in the knee. A randomized trial. J Bone Joint Surg Am 2004;86A(3):455–64.

[44] Gross AE. Repair of cartilage defects in the knee. J Knee Surg 2002;15(3):167–9.

[45] Mandelbaum BR, Browne JE, Fu F, Micheli L, Mosely Jr JB, Erggelet C, et al. Articular cartilage lesions of the knee. Am J Sports Med 1998;26(6):853–61.

[46] Cain EL, Clancy WG. Treatment algorithm for osteochondral injuries of the knee. Clin Sports Med 2001;20(2):321–42.

[47] Alleyne KR, Galloway MT. Management of osteochondral injuries of the knee. Clin Sports Med 2001;20(2):343–64.

[48] Messner K, Maletius W. The long-term prognosis for severe damage to weight-bearing cartilage in the knee. Acta Orthop Scand 1996;67:165–8.

ELSEVIER
SAUNDERS

Clin Sports Med 24 (2005) 175–186

CLINICS
IN SPORTS
MEDICINE

Sports after Total Joint Replacement

Phillip E. Clifford, MD, William J. Mallon, MD*

Triangle Orthopaedic Associates, 120 William Penn Plaza, Durham, NC 27704, USA

The development of joint replacement has improved the quality of life for millions of individuals worldwide. Decades ago, replacements were reserved for the inactive elderly. This subjected the implants to lower loads and fewer cycles of wear, leading to acceptable low rates of failure. The passage of the last 2 decades has brought numerous technologic advancements in implant designs and component manufacturing. These advances have allowed surgeons to offer total joint replacement to several new groups of patients with guarded successful outcomes in most cases [1–3]. These groups of patients include the very young active patients suffering posttraumatic osteoarthritis, the aging athlete who would prefer to continue "working out" as much as possible, the morbidly obese yet younger, active patient, the "baby-boomer" generation, and the elderly patients who continue to advance the average life expectancy while going to their second, third, and fourth revision total joints in an effort to maintain their cardiovascular health and remain active [4–7] (Figs. 1–5).

For most patients, the pain and decrease in activity level or lifestyle remain the central issues that help drive them to proceed with replacement surgery. After careful counseling by the operative surgeon to assist in understanding their postoperative expectations and restrictions, most patients in advanced discomfort with significant limitations decide to proceed with surgery. What seems to vary extensively in the literature and from surgeon to surgeon, is exactly what those restrictions should be for a given procedure. Once function has been restored and pain relieved, often patients break these restrictions and "abuse" their implants, creating increased risk of failure and loosening. We provide a rough guide to activity after joint replacement in an effort to stratify the risks of certain activities

---

* Corresponding author.

E-mail address: bmallon@nc.rr.com (W.J. Mallon).

0278-5919/05/$ – see front matter © 2004 Elsevier Inc. All rights reserved.
doi:10.1016/j.csm.2004.08.009

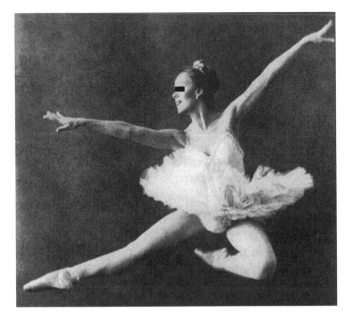

Fig. 1. A ballet dancer who continues to perform her sport after total hip replacement.

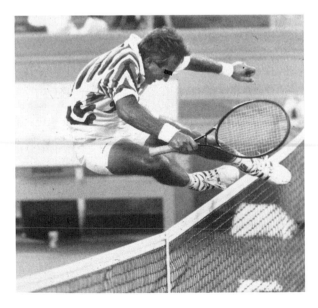

Fig. 2. Senior professional tennis player, formerly ranked #5 in the world, who continues to compete with bilateral total hip replacements. Caution: this man is a trained professional—we do not recommend you try this at home.

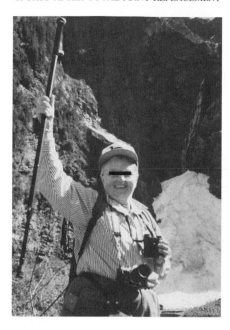

Fig. 3. Older woman who continues to hike multiple mountains in both the eastern and western United States after contralateral total hip and total knee replacements.

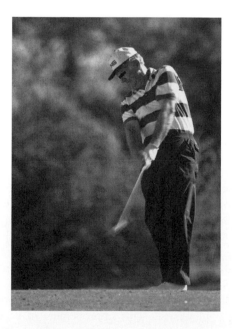

Fig. 4. Senior professional golfer, competing in the US Senior Open after bilateral total knee replacements.

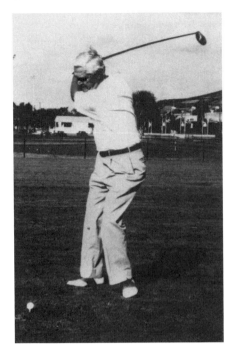 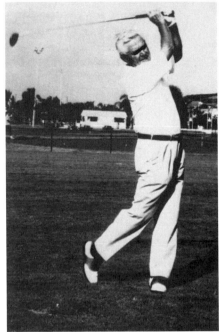

Fig. 5. Senior professional golfer, who continues to compete after bilateral total hip replacements.

for patients. This can allow patients to be as informed about their postoperative activity and its risks as their surgery itself.

Hip replacement

Hip replacement surgery has been the proving ground for technology, including new crosslinked wear-resistant plastics, durable less brittle ceramics, and precise micron-level metallurgy. Old avenues of thought that failed in the past are being reexplored, reinvented, and revisited. With our new technology and advances in manufacturing blending with our knowledge of past failures from the last 20 years, we hope to have three effective options for wear resistant bearing surfaces. The traditional failure in hip replacement surgery was typically osteolysis related to polyethylene wear and debris [8,9]. New crosslinked polyethylene liners seem to have negligible wear in hip simulators and early retrieval studies [10]. Durable plastics have led to larger head sizes, as wear is now much less of an issue. This increase in head size, coupled with a decrease in femoral stem neck diameter, has increased the range of motion in the standard hip replacement before impingement. This improvement in head–neck ratio along with routine standard capsular repair has decreased the rate of dislocation to levels near zero in several studies [11,12].

Other patients, typically younger and more active, are offered other options such as metal-on-metal and ceramic-on-ceramic implants. The newest versions of both of these implants seem to function well, although most current models lack long-term in vivo follow-up. Ceramic implants have fracture and subsequent third body wear as their only significant risks, and these are almost eliminated with the newest ceramics [13,14]. Metallic couples of both standard and resurfacing subtypes have the unknown risk of the metal ions and as well as microscopic debris. The Swedish Hip Registry continues to follow patients who have undergone metal-on-metal implant replacements from more than 20 years ago without obvious complication. Resurfacing techniques have gained favor with younger patients as they allow more activity including higher impact loading and a near normal range of motion, while conserving bone stock on both sides of the joint [15,16]. The anterior approach is recommended for resurfacing to preserve blood supply, and can lead to a more significant and longer lasting limp postoperatively.

Minimally invasive techniques and limited incision surgery has also allowed earlier return to activities after replacement surgery. The use of intraoperative fluoroscopy and specially designed retractors has reduced surgical dissection and decreased recovery times for patients [17].

Knee replacement

Numerous developments and improved partial replacements have emerged in recent years. Just as we are revisiting old ideas in hip replacement, partial knee replacements have experienced an intensive resurgence. The smaller incision and quick recovery compared with total replacement make these devices quite marketable. More recently, the limited incision has been applied to total replacements in an effort to improve recovery time and reduce the intensive physical therapy necessary in the postoperative period. In patients with osteoarthritis that remains limited to one compartment, unicompartmental replacement is favored by numerous surgeons [3]. Partial unispacer replacements of the medial compartment are performed with good success in appropriate candidates. This device glides between the denuded cartilage surfaces and can provide significant pain relief. For more advanced angular deformities or advance cystic arthritic changes, formal fixed unicompartmental components are best suited to improve the function of the joint. Recently, a new device that replaces the patellofemoral articular surface had been produced, and has had acceptable early results. Other surgeons remain cautious of partial replacements, as they can provide inadequate relief in patients with under appreciated, more advanced than expected, osteoarthritis. The complete replacement has experienced advances as well, such as rotating platform components, medial pivot tibial inserts, improved cruciate sparing designs and even crosslinked liners for the tibial component in an effort to minimize "back-side" wear of the tibial component [18–20].

Shoulder replacement

Shoulder arthroplasty has been an area of recent improvements in implant designs. Near custom implants and recreation of anatomic orientation has become possible with several designs of implants. Hemiarthroplasty and total shoulder replacements have each demonstrated excellent success in the correct clinical setting. Glenoid replacement has been the primary component of concern regarding possible loosening while humeral fixation with either cement or pressfit fixation has proven to be effective. Rotator cuff condition preoperatively plays a large role in eventual functional recovery. Patients with excellent cuff strength returned to more normal activities. Most shoulder surgeons will allow return to sports, especially golf, although limitations are more frequent in advanced overhead activities [21,22].

Elbow replacement

Constrained or linked hinged elbow arthroplasty remains the standard replacement for the elbow such as the Coonrad-Morrey. Recovery to the level of advanced participation in sports is rare, and can lead to loosening due to the constrained nature of the implants. Limiting activities to those of daily living is best for most patients, as anecdotal evidence suggests that elevated levels of function and forces leads to early loosening of the implants [21,22].

Ankle replacement

Recent advances in ankle replacement designs have led to improved results and lower failure rates. However, these improved results are similar to the early results with hip and knee replacements that were initially successful due in part to their use in the low demand population of the elderly less active patient. The newer designs are entering the early (3–8 year) stage results with surprisingly low loosening and failure rates [23]. Time and further advances will hopefully allow a more normal functional recovery after ankle replacement in the future, but for now, any significant impact weight bearing exercise is discouraged [22].

Discussion

Literature reviews on sport participation after replacement surgery are limited in number and scope, and based more on personal opinion rather than prospective studies. Lower impact exercise seems better tolerated by patients, and in theory, is less likely to create an environment for loosening whether it is secondary to wear debris osteolysis or impact-related loosening or a combination of both. As impact loading and torsional loading escalate, the relative risk associated with an activity increases. Presurgical activity and ability is also crucial to determine appropriate postsurgical activities. An example would be that a patient who have been downhill skiing all their life is more apt to tolerate that activity after replacement surgery with fewer complications than a patient who tries to learn to ski after surgery. The relative risk to the experienced patient may be theoretically less despite the fact that downhill skiing is a near high-risk activity.

Returning to a competitive sport after joint replacement is extremely difficult, as has been seen in the public eye as professional athletes over the last few decades have tried to accomplish this feat unsuccessfully. Recreational sports remain a similar challenge for most patients depending in large part on the stability and strength of their joint preoperatively. High levels of activity involving repetitive motions of a given sport were able to wear out the original joint. Any surgeon who believes his or her replacement joint can handle more forces than the original model should seriously reconsider their thinking. However, pre- and postoperative education are essential to helping each patient to choose their own exercise routine after replacement surgery.

Tables 1 and 2 contain information and recommendations concerning specific activities after joint arthroplasty surgery, based both on the location of the arthroplasty and the demand level for the activity [24–26].

Standard outcome studies for replacement surgery are too numerous to count when the literature is searched. However, the outcome of replacement surgery and return to sport has not been well studied. Most studies are retrospective and somewhat limited to anecdotal results that are inadequate for broad application across all patient populations [22,27–38]. Numerous authors have related increased failure rates to younger aged and more active patients. The most available data remains from hip replacement series, where we have learned that increased cycles of use leads to increased wear of the bearing surface. It is uncertain whether this previously accepted fact is, indeed, still truly a fact. Our newest crosslinked plastic bearing surfaces seem to show negligible wear after more than 27 million cycles in hip simulators. The metal and ceramic couples show no wear. We must then ask whether the bearing surface remains the weak link in the arthroplasty construct. If the attachment to bone then is the weak link and particulate debris has been all but removed from the equation, then how can the attachment be improved?

Wolfe's Law of bone simply put is "you use it or lose it." Weight-bearing exercise in the setting of well-fixed, in-grown components may actually be beneficial to the life of the implant. Herein lies the dilemma: how much is too much exercise, and how much impact loading is acceptable?

The type of sport and the extent of participation regarding competitive level and repetitive nature of movements is crucial. Those most important factors are the frequency of repetitive motions, the magnitude of joint loading, and the potential for falls and contact. The most serious of these is the latter, as significant contact or falls can cause catastrophic failure, dislocation, or fracture of bone or implants.

Table 1
Sports participation for patients with joint replacements based upon level of impact loading

Level of impact	Examples	Recommendations
Low	Stationary cycling Calisthenics Golf Stationary skiing Swimming Walking Ballroom dancing Water aerobics	Can improve general health Desirable for most patients, but may increase rate of wear Orthotics and activity modifications can reduce impact loads Concentration on conditioning and flexibility rather than strengthening
Potentially low	Bowling Fencing Rowing Isokinetic weight lifting Sailing Speed walking Crosscountry skiing Table tennis Jazz dancing and ballet Bicycling	Desirable for most patients, but may increase rate of wear Requires preactivity evaluation, monitoring, and development of guidelines by surgeon Balance and proprioception must be intact Orthotics and activity modifications can reduce impact loads Emphasize high number of repetitions with minimal resistance
Intermediate	Free weight lifting Hiking Horseback riding Ice skating Rock climbing Low-impact aerobics Tennis In-line skating Downhill skiing	Appropriate only for selected patients Require preactivity evaluation, monitoring, and development of guidelines for participation by surgeon Excellent physical condition is necessary Orthotics, impact absorbing shoes and activity modification frequently necessary
High	Baseball/softball Basketball/volleyball Football Handball/racketball Jogging/running Lacrosse Soccer Water skiing Karate	Should be avoided Significant probability of injury and need for revision

The frequency and magnitude of repetitive impact loading remains extremely controversial. At a recent conference of hip replacement specialists, a videotape was shown of a patient who continues to run status postceramic-on-ceramic hip replacement. His mileage is 7 to 9 miles three to five times a week. The presenting surgeon was criticized for proudly displaying his patient's "abuse" of his implant. Although we have no control over our patients after their replacement, we can learn from their indiscretions. If this patient's implants remain well fixed and show improved in-growth radiographically, and if his ceramic bearing does not fracture under repeated impact, will that change our future restrictions for our young active patients?

Table 2
Sports participation for patients with joint replacements based upon anatomic location of arthroplasty

Sport	Acceptable	Possible	Not recommended
Ballet dancing	Shoulder	Hip, knee	
Ballroom dancing	Hip, Knee, Shoulder		
Baseball/softball			Hip, knee, shoulder
Basketball			Hip, knee, shoulder
Bicycling	Hip, knee, shoulder		
Bowling	Hip, knee	Shoulder	
Calisthenics		Hip, knee, shoulder	
Crosscountry skiing	Hip, knee, shoulder		
Downhill skiing	Shoulder	Hip, knee	
Fencing		Hip, knee	Shoulder
Football			Hip, knee, shoulder
Golf	Hip, knee, shoulder		
Handball/racketball		Shoulder	Hip, knee
Hiking	Shoulder	Hip, knee	
Horseback riding	Hip, knee, shoulder		
Ice skating	Hip, knee, shoulder		
In-line skating	Hip, knee, shoulder		
Jazz dancing	Shoulder	Hip, knee	
Jogging/running	Shoulder	Hip, knee	
Karate			Hip, knee, shoulder
Lacrosse			Hip, knee, shoulder
Low-impact aerobics	Hip, knee, shoulder		
Rock climbing		Hip, knee, shoulder	
Rowing	Hip, knee	Shoulder	
Sailing	Hip, knee, shoulder		
Soccer		Shoulder	Hip, knee
Speed walking	Hip, knee, shoulder		
Stationary cycling	Hip, knee, shoulder		
Stationary skiing	Hip, knee, shoulder		
Swimming	Hip, knee	Shoulder	
Table tennis		Hip, knee, shoulder	
Tennis		Hip, knee, shoulder	
Volleyball			Hip, knee, shoulder
Walking	Hip, knee, shoulder		
Water aerobics	Hip, knee, shoulder		
Water skiing		Hip, knee	Shoulder
Weight lifting			

Golf remains the best studied activity after joint replacement. These studies are retrospective, but can help with guidelines for return to sport [22,32,33]. Most golfers do experience some discomfort after playing golf following hip or knee replacement surgery. Hip replacements are better tolerated overall than knee replacements. Right-handed golfers had more difficulty with left knee replacements than with right knee replacements [22,32,33].

Low-impact sports including stationary cycling, dancing, golf, stationary skiing, swimming, and walking are tolerated the best with the fewest symptoms. Bowling, fencing, weight training, sailing, rowing, speed walking, and crosscountry skiing are also tolerated well, although do have more impact potential and increased joint reaction forces that equates to wear rates. This group of activities remains universally accepted by surgeons [30,35].

Intermediate impact loading activities such as bicycling, hiking, horseback riding, ice skating, rock climbing, in-line skating, doubles tennis, and downhill skiing are possible after replacement surgery [30,35]. Patients who have participated in these activities with a degree of proficiency before their replacement surgery can likely return to that activity at a slightly lower level of function. Conditioning before return to sport should be guided toward adequate muscle strengthening and conditioning to allow a return to the highest level of participation in that sport with the least risk. Avoiding suboptimal conditions helps avoid injuries. Tennis should not be played on wet surfaces. Downhill skiers should avoid steep ungroomed runs and moguls and concentrate on well-groomed wide runs without icy conditions.

Most surgeons strongly discourage high-impact loading sports such as softball, football, basketball, racquetball, running, singles tennis, soccer, water skiing, and impact karate [30,35]. The consequences of engaging in the activities can result in major complications. The need for further surgery with predictably poorer outcomes than primary replacements is a real risk. Revision surgery can present significant challenges to the operative surgeon, and can significantly impact functional recovery potential.

Most patients can return to low- to intermediate-impact activities within 3 to 6 months following replacement. Crucial to their return is the postsurgical therapy and their preoperative ability. Gradually returning to previous levels of activity is essential. Patients must avoid overworking a joint that has not had adequate time to strengthen itself to a level so that the muscles around the joint can "share the load." Each patient must understand that their success and recovery cannot be measured against other patients or even against their own prior replacement experience. Each patient and each joint can differ greatly in their recovery time table.

Summary

Today's patients require additional guidance in their expectations after replacement surgery. Failure rates for shoulder, hip, and knee, replacements across most studies are approximately 0.5% to 1% per year, including infection, loosening, and wear of the parts. Elbow and ankle replacements will likely require more restrictions and have slightly higher revision rates.

As the aging population of "weekend warriors" tries to maintain their fitness craze of the seventies and eighties, another segment of the population "super-sizes" themselves into morbid obesity. The increasing life expectancy of the elderly and their need for revision surgery coupled with the population expanse of the baby-boomer generation makes for a very busy future in replacement surgery. As each of these groups try to push the durability and longevity of the current-day implants to the limit by maintaining active lifestyles that repetitively cycle the implants or repetitively cycles the implants with excessive loads, we will realize the limitations of our new technologies and interventions and possibly better learn what to recommend to our patients in the future.

References

[1] Burroughs PL, Gearen PF, Petty WR, Wright TW. Shoulder arthroplasty in the young patient. J Arthroplasty 2003;18(6):792–8.

[2] Keener JD, Callaghan JJ, Goetz DD, Pederson DR, Sullivan PM, Johnston RC. Twenty-five year results after Charnley total hip arthroplasty in patients less than fifty years old. J Bone Joint Surg 2003;85-A(6):1066–72.

[3] Pennington DW, Swienckowski JJ, Lutes WB, Drake GN. Unicompartmental knee arthroplasty in patients sixty years of age or younger. J Bone Joint Surg 2003;85-A(10):1968–73.

[4] Gidwani S, Tauro B, Whitehouse S, Newman JH. Do patients need to earn total knee arthroplasty? J Arthroplasty 2003;18(2):199–203.

[5] Felson DT. Epidemiology of hip and knee osteoarthritis. Epidemiol Rev 1988;10:1–28.

[6] Garrick JG, Requa RK. Sports fitness activities: the negative consequences. J Am Acad Orthop Surg 2003;11:439–43.

[7] Ashe MC, Khan KM. Exercise prescription. J Am Acad Orthop Surg 2004;12:21–7.

[8] Harris WH. Osteolysis and particle disease in hip replacement: a review. Acta Orthop Scand 1994;65:113–23.

[9] Chew FS, Lev MH. Polyethylene osteolysis. Am J Roentgenol 1992;159:1254–7.

[10] Muratoglu OK, Greenbaum ES, Bragdon CR, Jasty M, Freiberg AA, Harris WM. Surface analysis of early retrieved acetabular polyethylene liners: a comparison of conventional and highly crosslinked polyethylenes. J Arthroplasty 2004;19(1):68–77.

[11] Weeden SH, Paprosky WG, Bowling J. The early dislocation rate in primary total hip arthroplasty following the posterior approach with posterior soft tissue repair. J Arthroplasty 2003;18(6):709–13.

[12] Pellici PM, Bostrom M, Poss R. Posterior approach to total hip replacement using enhanced posterior soft tissue repair. Clin Orthop 1998;355:224–8.

[13] Ranawat CS, Padgett DE, Ohashi Y. Total knee arthroplasty for patients younger than 55. Clin Orthop 1989;248:27–33.

[14] Stewart TD, Tipper JL, Streicher RM, Ingham E, Fisher J. Severe wear and fracture of zirconia heads against alumina inserts in hip simulator studies with microseparation. J Arthroplasty 2003;18(6):726–34.

[15] Amstutz HC, Beavle PE, Dorey FU, et al. Metal-on-metal hybrid surface arthroplasty: two to six year follow-up study. J Bone Joint Surg 2004;86-A(1):28–39.

[16] Silva M, Lee KH, Heisel C, Dela Rosa MA, Schmalzried TP. The biomechanical results of total hip resurfacing arthroplasty. J Bone Joint Surg 2004;86-A(1):40–6.

[17] DiGioia AM, Plakseychuk AY, Levison TJ, et al. Mini-incision technique for total hip arthroplasty with navigation. J Arthroplasty 2003;18(2):123–8.

[18] Akisue T, Yamaguchi M, Bauer TW, et al. "Backside" polyethylene deformation in total knee arthroplasty. J Arthroplasty 2003;18(6):784–91.

[19] Malhotra R. Results of rotating-platform low-contact stress knee prosthesis. J Arthroplasty 2003; 18(8):1016–22.

[20] Oakeshott R, Stiehl JB, Komistek RA, et al. Kinematic analysis of a posterior cruciate re-taining mobile bearing total knee arthroplasty. J Arthroplasty 2003;18(8):1029–37.

[21] Collis DK. Degenerative diseases and golf. In: The neck, shoulder and upper extremities in sports (and special golf panel). Eugene (OR): Postgraduate Course of the American Academy of Orthopaedic Surgeons; July 1974. p. 78–87.

[22] Mallon WJ. Total joint replacement and golf. In: McCarroll JR, Stover CS, Mallon WJ, editors. Medical aspects of golf. Philadelphia: FA Davis; 1992. p. 85–94.

[23] Anderson T, Montgomery F, Carlsson A. Uncemented STAR total ankle prosthesis. Three to eight year follow-up of fifty-one consecutive ankles. J Bone Joint Surg 2003;85-A(7):1321–9.

[24] Mallon WJ, Liebelt RA, Mason JB. Total joint replacement and golf. Clin Sports Med 1996; 15(1):179–90.

[25] Vail TP, Mallon WJ, Liebelt RA. Athletic activities after joint arthroplasty. Sports Med Arthroscopy Rev 1996;4:298–305.

[26] Mallon WJ, Vail TP. Sport after total joint arthroplasty. In: Maffulli N, Chan K-M, Macdonald R, Malina RM, Parker AQ, editors. Sports medicine for specific ages and abilities. Edinburgh: Churchill Livingstone; 2001. p. 307–14.

[27] Andriacchi TP, Galante JO, Fermier RW. The influence of total knee arthroplasty design on walking and stair climbing. J Bone Joint Surg 1982;64-B:1328–35.

[28] Dubs L, Gschwend N, Munzinger U, et al. Sport after total hip arthroplasty. Arch Orthop Traumat Surg 1983;101:161–9.

[29] Kilgus DJ, Dorey FJ, Finerman GAM, Amstutz HC. Patient activity, sports participation, and impact loading on the durability of cemented total hip replacements. Clin Orthop 1991;269: 25–31.

[30] McGrory BJ, Stuart MJ, Sim FH. Participation in sports after hip and knee arthroplasty: review of the literature and survey of surgeon preferences. Mayo Clin Proc 1995;70:342–8.

[31] MacNicol MF, McHardy R, Chalmers J. Exercise testing before and after hip arthroplasty. J Bone Joint Surg 1980;62-B:326–31.

[32] Mallon WJ, Callaghan JJ. Total hip replacement in active golfers. J Arthroplasty 1992;7(Suppl): 339–46.

[33] Mallon WJ, Callaghan JJ. Total knee participation in active golfers. J Arthroplasty 1993;8: 299–306.

[34] Minns RJ, Crawford RJ, Porter ML, Hardinge K. Muscle strength following total hip arthroplasty: a comparison of trochanteric osteotomy and the direct lateral approach. J Arthroplasty 1993;8:625–7.

[35] Ritter MA, Meding JB. Total hip arthroplasty: can the patient play sports again? Orthopaedics 1987;10:1447–52.

[36] Stiehl JB, deAndrade JR. Activities after replacement of the hip and knee. Orthopaedics 1995; 1:32–3.

[37] Visuri T, Nonkanen R. Total hip replacment: its influence on spontaneous recreation exercise habits. Arch Phys Med Rehabil 1980;61:325–8.

[38] White J. No more bump and grind. Phys Sportsmed 1992;20:223–8.

ELSEVIER
SAUNDERS

CLINICS
IN SPORTS
MEDICINE

Clin Sports Med 24 (2005) 187–198

Impact of Osteoarthritis on Sports Careers

Brian R. Wolf, MD*, Annunziato Amendola, MD

*Department of Orthopaedics and Rehabilitation, University of Iowa Sports Medicine,
200 Hawkins Drive, Iowa City, IA 52242, USA*

It is not uncommon to open the sports page in the newspaper and find an article of an established professional athlete whose career has been "cut short" for medical reasons. In many cases that reason is the development of joint arthritis that limits that athlete's ability to compete at their former level. Relatively recent examples have included a former Super Bowl most valuable player running back and a starting first baseman for a major league baseball team. This occurrence is likely even more common among current or former amateur athletes, including those in college and high school. In addition, a compounding factor increasing the prevalence of injury is that overall, participation in sports has exploded over the last few decades. In the United States, this has been especially true in sports with high risks of injury such as soccer and women's basketball [1–3]. Participation in load-bearing and impact sports places competitors at risk of suffering injuries, usually to the lower extremities. Even in the absence of injury, repetitive joint overuse is the likely cause of osteoarthritis (OA) in many current and former athletes [4,5]. The purpose of this article is to explore and summarize what is known, and what is not yet known, regarding the relationship of OA and sports participation on all levels.

Osteoarthritis

OA is the progressive loss of normal cartilage structure and function [5,6]. It involves all the tissues of the joint, including the bone, capsule, synovium, and the cartilage [7]. During any review of the literature regarding OA, it is important

---

* Corresponding author.
E-mail address: brian-wolf@uiowa.edu (B.R. Wolf).

to understand how it is being defined [8]. Clinical exam, radiographs, arthroscopic changes, patient complaints, and symptoms are often used to monitor and assess for OA. The joints that commonly become arthritic in the general population are the hip, knee, lumbar and cervical spine, and base of the thumb, all of which are involved in load bearing [8]. Most often the process of OA begins with disruption of the superficial layer of cartilage that grossly appears as diffuse or localized fibrillation [5]. This is associated with decreased proteoglycan concentration and increased water content in the cartilage. With time, and continued mechanical insult, the fibrillation can progress to fissures and cracks that penetrate deeper into the cartilage, with degenerative change eventually reaching the level of the subchondral bone. The amount of cartilage lost relates to continued degeneration and fragmentation of all cartilage layers after the development of clefts. Enzymatic degradation also occurs, reducing cartilage volume [5–7]. The process of OA is also associated with an inflammatory aspect that is evidenced by positive bone scans, synovitis, and elevated serum markers such as C-reactive protein [9,10]. Such markers have been used to mark the progression of OA in addition to standard radiographs and clinical exam.

Risk factors for osteoarthritis

There are multiple risk factors for OA; many that are known, some that are impossible to measure, and likely some factors that have yet to be appreciated. Among those generally agreed upon risk factors for OA are general/systemic variables such as age, gender, and genetic predisposition [8]. In addition, biomechanical factors such as knee alignment, obesity, and knee injury or trauma are very important as well [5,8]. One of the problems in trying to relate exercise and sport with subsequent OA is accounting for occupational risks and exposures in people who are not professional athletes [8]. For example, high levels of hip and knee OA have been associated with jobs requiring repetitive heavy lifting, kneeling, and squatting [11–13]. Determining whether OA is due to sports participation or other factors for an athlete is difficult at best.

Joint injury seems to be a consistent risk factor for possible subsequent joint OA. One large series has suggested that a history of joint injury increases the incidence rate of joint OA but does not affect the rate of progression of OA [14]. From the Swedish registries, Vingard found that in the group that reported a history of the highest sports participation, over 800 hours in total, men and women had relative risks of developing hip OA requiring total joint replacement of 4.5 and 2.3 compared with the lowest sports participation groups [15,16]. Interestingly, those men that had also been employed with a heavy labor job with high joint-loading activities, combined with a history of high levels of sports participation, had a relative risk nearly double those who worked in nonheavy labor jobs. Lane reported on the finding of a regression analysis on predictors of hip OA in a series of 5818 women with a mean age of 72 [17]. Those women who reported higher levels of recreational activities as teenagers, at age 30 and at age 50, had significantly higher odds of moderate to severe hip OA compared with those who reported no recreational activities. Obviously, studies such as these are limited by recall bias of symptomatic patients.

Another difficult issue for all of these studies is distinguishing the relationship of high loading sports and subsequent OA when a major confounder is the history of joint injury in the past [8]. Joint injury can be a single impact load that acutely causes articular cartilage damage [5]. Yet, it can also be due to repetitive micro-trauma during sports participation that can lead to splits and fissures in articular cartilage [5,18], because cartilage is aneural subtle damage, and injury can be imparted on joint surfaces without symptoms occurring in athletes [5]. In an extensively matched case–control study by Sutton et al, 216 patients with reported knee OA and four controls per patient were extensively questioned regarding lifetime exercise participation [19]. The only risk factor that was found to be significant was a history of a prior knee injury, which had an odds ratio of 8.0.

A significant percentage of joint injuries occur during sports and related activities. More data is becoming available evaluating injury rates with specific sports. For example, in elite soccer players injury rates of 6.8 to 8.5 per 1000 hours of participation have been found, with injuries more common during games than during training, and approximately 20% being recurrent injuries [20,21]. The long-term importance of joint injury and the risk for subsequent OA has been confirmed in large prospective cohort studies [14,22]. In the lower extremity, meniscal tears, chondral injuries, and anterior cruciate ligament (ACL) tears are associated with both contact and noncontact mechanisms, often related to a twisting or pivoting episode of the lower extremity (Fig. 1). Studies that have linked meniscal injuries, ligament tears, and articular fractures with subsequent OA have often been based on sports participation [23–27]. In studies that have evaluated the long-term outcomes of arthroscopic partial meniscectomy,

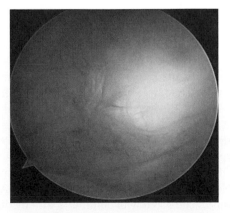

Fig. 1. Symptomatic anterior lateral tibial plateau lesion with grade 2 to 3 changes in a 21-year-old female basketball player following a hyperextension knee injury associated with a posterior cruciate ligament tear.

approximately 50% of patients have been found to have some radiographic signs of OA at 8 to 12 years [28,29]. Similarly, high rates of OA in have been documented in knees with a history of an ACL tear, regardless of whether a reconstruction was performed or not [23]. In the upper extremity a shoulder dislocation is often associated with sports participation. Using a case–control analysis Marx et al found that a prior shoulder dislocation increased the risk of subsequent shoulder OA 10 to 20 times that of an uninjured shoulder [30].

Sport type and osteoarthritis

The type of sport is an important factor regarding the subsequent risk for OA, with high-impact sports being more detrimental. A study on 2000 former elite international athletes that competed in endurance (running, crosscountry skiing), team (soccer, hockey, basketball) or power sports (boxing, wrestling, weight lifting) was performed, using over 20 years of data on subsequent hospital admissions for diagnoses related to hip, knee, or ankle OA [31–33]. All three groups had increased rates of OA compared with the control group, with the team and power athletes having the highest rates. Radiographic evidence of knee OA among 117 of these athletes was found in 31% of weight lifters, 29% of soccer players, 14% of long-distance runners, and 3% of shooters [32]. This increased risk was related to increased injury risk in the soccer players and increased body mass index at age 20 in the weight lifters. Subsequent hip and knee disability among these athletes was also examined [33]. Power sport competitors had the highest odds ratio for hip disability. High risk of knee disability was only seen among the team sports participants, again likely reflecting the increased risk of injury in certain sports.

For sports such as running, where there is less chance of injury, there exists some controversy on the role of exercise and the subsequent risk of OA. Marti et al looked at the effect of excessive running on rates of hip OA [34]. This study was a retrospective cohort that reported on examinations that were done in 1973 and in 1988 on 27 long-distance runners who averaged 60 miles per week in 1973. The control groups were nine bobsleigh riders and 23 controls. In 1988, at average age of 42, radiographic evidence of hip OA was found in 19% of the runners and in neither of the other two groups. The two predictive factors were miles run per week in 1973 and age. Radiographic hip and knee OA was also evaluated in 67 elite middle and long-distance runners, female tennis players, and a matched control group in a study by Spector et al [35]. Hip and knee OA were significantly higher in the athletes with runners having more patellofemoral OA.

Several studies have, however, produced different conclusions regarding running and OA. No difference in rates of radiographic OA were found in 60 former marathon runners compared with controls in a study done in 1975 [36]. In a small prospective study of 17 runners, no difference in rates of radiographic OA of the hip, knee, ankle, or foot OA were found compared with a control group [37]. Lane et al have published on a long-distance running club over a prospective period of time monitoring rates of OA. A group of 41 club runners were found at baseline to have similar rates of knee and spine OA compared with matched controls [38]. Runners and controls subsequently had similar rates of knee OA at 5- and 9-year follow-ups [39,40]. Hip OA was also found to be no different between the groups at 9 years. Regression analysis for the runners revealed that baseline radiographic score and pace of running were predictors of OA. Last, a final study matching 30 distance runners with controls found no difference in rates of radiographic OA of the hips, knees, and ankles for a group of runners who averaged between 12 and 25 miles per week over a median age of 40 [41].

Follow-up studies have also been done evaluating OA in other individual sports, in some cases showing increased rates of upper extremity OA. AC joint arthrosis has been associated with history of high physical workload and sports. A relative risk of 5.0 and 3.0 for developing AC joint OA on the right and left sides, respectively, was found for those participating in high-level sports compared with low-level sports [42]. Increased hand OA has been found in rock climbers. Radiographs of the hands of 36 rock climbers were compared with matched controls, with evidence of radiographic OA found in 17 of the rock climbers and only two of the controls [43]. Among throwing sports only javelin throwers have been evaluated for subsequent joint OA problems. Twenty-one elite javelin throwers were evaluated for shoulder and elbow arthritis at a mean of 19 years after completion of participation [44]. Five athletes complained of transient shoulder pain and three complained of transient elbow pain. Magnetic resonance imaging (MRI) revealed increased numbers of rotator cuff tears in the dominant arm compared with the nonthrowing arm. In addition, all of these athletes had radiographic evidence of elbow OA and 10 lacked at least 5 degrees of elbow extension compared with the nondominant limb. In a separate study elite javelin throwers and high jumpers were also found to have higher incidence of radiographic hip OA at least 10 years after retirement compared with controls [45].

Among team sports, soccer is one of the most frequently studied due to its worldwide popularity. A retrospective analysis of 215 nonelite and 71 elite former soccer players evaluated signs of hip and knee radiographic OA compared with age-matched controls [46,47]. The elite players had a 14% rate of hip OA compared with 4.2% in the nonelite players and controls [47]. Evidence of radiographic knee OA was 15.5%, 4.2%, and 1.6% for the elite, nonelite, and control groups, respectively [46]. Hip OA has been found to be higher in soccer players despite no history of injury [48]. Other series have also reported rates of lower limb OA between 32% and 49% in former professional soccer players, with the knee being the most frequent site [49,50].

In Australian rules football, greater prevalence of radiographic and clinical knee arthritis was found in 50 footballers compared with controls, with a history of injury increasing the risk of OA [51]. Moderate to severe radiographic knee OA was found in 24% of the retired elite footballers compared with 6% of the control group. Functional OA was found in 25% of the footballers compared with 1% of the control group. Data on Australian rugby also suggests elevated percentages of radiographic and clinically significant OA of the knee [52]. Increased rates of radiographic OA changes have been found in 22 elite volleyball players who had played at least 3 years in the elite volleyball league in Switzerland compared with controls [53]. No good studies have been done to evaluate the rates of radiographic or clinical osteoarthritis in the popular American sports such as baseball, basketball, or football.

The impact of joint osteoarthritis

The effects of OA changes in different joints in the body have different implications for participants in different sports. Arthritic changes of any of the lower extremity joints are going to be ill-tolerated for those participating in running, cutting, or pivoting sports such as basketball, football skill players, soccer, tennis, and so on. For professional players, development of OA in the lower extremity can hasten the end of their career. Despite long-term consequences, unless the player is a quarterback or their sport involves some overhead activity such as tennis, arthritic changes in the shoulder, elbow, wrist, hands likely will be well tolerated and not impact many athletes' career. On the contrary, overhead athletes such as tennis players, baseball players, swimmers, and football quarterbacks would be far less tolerant to OA changes involving the upper extremities, especially in the dominant arm. Last, just about any athlete's career or participation level can be drastically affected by any symptomatic OA changes in the spine. This is true of contact sports such as football and rugby, as well as noncontact low-impact sports such as golf.

It has been well documented that radiographic OA often does not correlate with a patient's or athlete's symptoms [54]. No literature exists for how different stages of OA affect athletes' performance or how long an athlete can compete with different lesions. In one study by Vertullo and Nunley involving a survey of

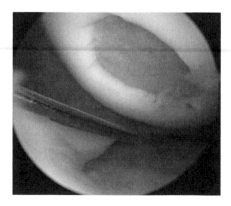

Fig. 2. A 27-year-old female with history of chronic anterior cruciate ligament tear suffered during participation in basketball in high school and this focal grade 4 lesion of the medial femoral condyle of unknown duration.

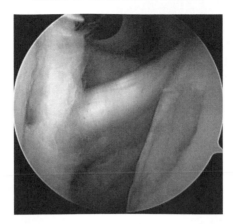

Fig. 3. A 40-year-old female that plays tennis three to five times a week with focal grade 3 to 4 lesion of the humeral head.

professional team physicians on the prevalence of players participating with fusions of the foot or ankle, no players were active with any hindfoot fusions, but there were some with metatarsophalangeal or tarsometatarsal joint fusions [55]. This study indicates that the joint involved and sport will determine if participation is possible in the presence of advanced OA. It is unknown how long an athlete in any sport can compete with untreated focal grade 4 changes, such as that in Figs. 2 and 3, or with grade 1 or 2 changes, such as those commonly seen on the patellar surface as seen in Fig. 4. Most would assume that focal grade 4 changes in the hip, knee, or ankle would cause pain, swelling, and problems for most athletes regardless of sport. However, we likely will never know the true answer because these lesions may be missed or may be minimally symptomatic in some individuals. Similarly, we assume that diffuse grade 2 or grade 3 changes may be extremely limiting, especially in the lower extremity joints in competitive

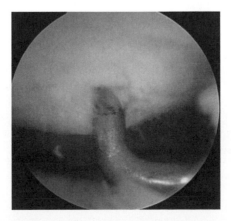

Fig. 4. Asymptomatic diffuse grade 2 chondromalacia changes on the patella in a 26-year-old runner who averages 25 to 30 miles a week. He also had a lateral meniscus tear and cyst.

athletes at all levels. But again, there likely are athletes that are minimally affected by these early OA changes and continue high levels of participation for long periods of time. It is likely that the location of the defect also plays a key role in whichever joint is affected, whether in the lower or upper extremity. A focal grade 4 lesion somewhere in the wrist or elbow may be disabling for a golfer, whereas diffuse hip grade 2 changes are well tolerated. This lack of clarity often makes counseling athletes with such lesions difficult. Accurately predicting their future sports function and ultimate outcome may be impossible.

Evaluating and monitoring osteoarthritis

Currently, the most common methods used to monitor incidence of and progression of OA are clinical examination and radiographs. However, previous studies have shown poor correlation between symptoms and joint damage as judged by radiographic evidence of OA [54]. New parameters to monitor OA are being developed. Newer imaging techniques with MRI have found associations between patient pain and bone edema and synovial hypertrophy [56–58]. MRI has been used to investigate subtle OA on cartilage-specific sequences changes likely not present on routine radiographs [59–61]. MRI investigations have also suggested the association of an acute injury with subsequent OA as well. Six years following anterior cruciate injury cartilage thinning was seen in a significant number of patients where previous osteochondral injury had been noted, and over half continued to have altered bone marrow edema [62]. There has also been interest in the use of biomarkers as indicators of OA. Techniques for this are being explored by several investigators, but their role and best use has not yet been clearly defined [63,64].

Benefits of sports and exercise

Although much of the data concludes that a risk of developing OA is related to exercise and sports participation, the long-term benefits of exercise should not be overshadowed. Lane found that 498 runners had better cardiovascular fitness and reduced obesity, and used medical services less often, compared with population controls [65]. Sarna reported a very large cohort of Finnish male elite athletes from the national registries [66]. Those athletes that had competed in aerobic type sports, team and endurance sports, had a long life expectance and low risks of ischemic heart disease and diabetes.

Summary

Overall, the literature would suggest that there is a higher risk of OA in both the lower extremity in sports participants in high joint loading and impact sports, and this risk is strongly associated with joint injury. On the contrary, moderate amounts of exercise for fitness appear to be safe and to not lead to OA. Similarly, in sports placing abnormal stress on joints in the upper extremity, increased rates of OA have also been found. In addition to sports participation, an athlete's body mass index, joint alignment, genetic predisposition, outside occupation, and other factors can influence the likelihood of subsequent joint OA. The specific joint that develops OA, as well as the specific location of OA in that joint, can have dramatically variable impacts on athletes in different sports. Further studies need to be completed to gain more information on specific sports participation, injury, and subsequent OA changes. This information would be invaluable in efforts to prevent joint disability in former athletes, and possibly to lengthen sports careers.

References

[1] Census UBot. Statistical abstract of the United States. 118th edition. Washington (DC): US Bureau of the Census; 1998.

[2] Census USBot. Statistical abstract of the United States: 1990. 110th edition. Washington (DC): US Bureau of the Census; 1990.

[3] Garrick JG, Requa RK. Sports and fitness activities: the negative consequences. J Am Acad Orthop Surg 2003;11(6):439–43.

[4] Lequesne MG, Dang N, Lane NE. Sport practice and osteoarthritis of the limbs. Osteoarthritis Cartilage 1997;5(2):75–86.

[5] Buckwalter JA, Lane NE. Athletics and osteoarthritis. Am J Sports Med 1997;25(6):873–81.

[6] Buckwalter JA, Martin J. Degenerative joint disease. Clin Symp 1995;47(2):1–32.

[7] Buckwalter JA, Mankin HJ. Articular cartilage: degeneration and osteoarthritis, repair, regeneration, and transplantation. Instr Course Lect 1998;47:487–504.

[8] Conaghan PG. Update on osteoarthritis part 1: current concepts and the relation to exercise. Br J Sports Med 2002;36(5):330–3.

[9] Ayral X, Ravaud P, Bonvarlet JP, et al. Arthroscopic evaluation of post-traumatic patellofemoral chondropathy. J Rheumatol 1999;26(5):1140–7.

[10] Kirwan JR, Elson CJ. Is the progression of osteoarthritis phasic? Evidence and implications. J Rheumatol 2000;27(4):834–6.

[11] McAlindon TE, Wilson PW, Aliabadi P, Weissman B, Felson DT. Level of physical activity and the risk of radiographic and symptomatic knee osteoarthritis in the elderly: the Framingham study. Am J Med 1999;106(2):151–7.

[12] Maetzel A, Makela M, Hawker G, Bombardier C. Osteoarthritis of the hip and knee and mechanical occupational exposure—a systematic overview of the evidence. J Rheumatol 1997; 24(8):1599–607.

[13] Coggon D, Croft P, Kellingray S, Barrett D, McLaren M, Cooper C. Occupational physical activities and osteoarthritis of the knee. Arthritis Rheum 2000;43(7):1443–9.

[14] Cooper C, Snow S, McAlindon TE, et al. Risk factors for the incidence and progression of radiographic knee osteoarthritis. Arthritis Rheum 2000;43(5):995–1000.

[15] Vingard E, Alfredsson L, Goldie I, Hogstedt C. Sports and osteoarthrosis of the hip. An epidemiologic study. Am J Sports Med 1993;21(2):195–200.

[16] Vingard E, Alfredsson L, Malchau H. Osteoarthrosis of the hip in women and its relationship to physical load from sports activities. Am J Sports Med 1998;26(1):78–82.

[17] Lane NE, Hochberg MC, Pressman A, Scott JC, Nevitt MC. Recreational physical activity and the risk of osteoarthritis of the hip in elderly women. J Rheumatol 1999;26(4):849–54.

[18] Dekel S, Weissman SL. Joint changes after overuse and peak overloading of rabbit knees in vivo. Acta Orthop Scand 1978;49(6):519–28.

[19] Sutton AJ, Muir KR, Mockett S, Fentem P. A case–control study to investigate the relation between low and moderate levels of physical activity and osteoarthritis of the knee using data collected as part of the Allied Dunbar National Fitness Survey. Ann Rheum Dis 2001; 60(8):756–64.

[20] Soderman K, Adolphson J, Lorentzon R, Alfredson H. Injuries in adolescent female players in European football: a prospective study over one outdoor soccer season. Scand J Med Sci Sports 2001;11(5):299–304.

[21] Hawkins RD, Fuller CW. A prospective epidemiological study of injuries in four English professional football clubs. Br J Sports Med 1999;33(3):196–203.

[22] Gelber AC, Hochberg MC, Mead LA, Wang NY, Wigley FM, Klag MJ. Joint injury in young adults and risk for subsequent knee and hip osteoarthritis. Ann Intern Med 2000;133(5):321–8.

[23] Gillquist J, Messner K. Anterior cruciate ligament reconstruction and the long-term incidence of gonarthrosis. Sports Med 1999;27(3):143–56.

[24] Honkonen SE. Degenerative arthritis after tibial plateau fractures. J Orthop Trauma 1995; 9(4):273–7.

[25] Lundberg M, Messner K. Ten-year prognosis of isolated and combined medial collateral ligament ruptures. A matched comparison in 40 patients using clinical and radiographic evaluations. Am J Sports Med 1997;25(1):2–6.

[26] Neyret P, Donell ST, DeJour D, DeJour H. Partial meniscectomy and anterior cruciate ligament rupture in soccer players. A study with a minimum 20-year followup. Am J Sports Med 1993; 21(3):455–60.

[27] Roos H, Lauren M, Adalberth T, Roos EM, Jonsson K, Lohmander LS. Knee osteoarthritis after meniscectomy: prevalence of radiographic changes after twenty-one years, compared with matched controls. Arthritis Rheum 1998;41(4):687–93.

[28] Fauno P, Nielsen AB. Arthroscopic partial meniscectomy: a long-term follow-up. Arthroscopy 1992;8(3):345–9.

[29] Higuchi H, Kimura M, Shirakura K, Terauchi M, Takagishi K. Factors affecting long-term results after arthroscopic partial meniscectomy. Clin Orthop 2000;377:161–8.

[30] Marx RG, McCarty EC, Montemurno TD, Altchek DW, Craig EV, Warren RF. Development of arthrosis following dislocation of the shoulder: a case–control study. J Shoulder Elbow Surg 2002;11(1):1–5.

[31] Kujala UM, Kaprio J, Sarna S. Osteoarthritis of weight bearing joints of lower limbs in former elite male athletes. Br Med J 1994;308(6923):231–4.

[32] Kujala UM, Kettunen J, Paananen H, et al. Knee osteoarthritis in former runners, soccer players, weight lifters, and shooters. Arthritis Rheum 1995;38(4):539–46.

[33] Kettunen JA, Kujala UM, Kaprio J, Koskenvuo M, Sarna S. Lower-limb function among former elite male athletes. Am J Sports Med 2001;29(1):2–8.

[34] Marti B, Knobloch M, Tschopp A, Jucker A, Howald H. Is excessive running predictive of degenerative hip disease? Controlled study of former elite athletes. Br Med J 1989; 299(6691):91–3.

[35] Spector TD, Harris PA, Hart DJ, et al. Risk of osteoarthritis associated with long-term weight-bearing sports: a radiologic survey of the hips and knees in female ex-athletes and population controls. Arthritis Rheum 1996;39(6):988–95.

[36] Puranen J, Ala-Ketola L, Peltokallio P, Saarela J. Running and primary osteoarthritis of the hip. Br Med J 1975;2(5968):424–5.

[37] Panush RS, Schmidt C, Caldwell JR, et al. Is running associated with degenerative joint disease? JAMA 1986;255(9):1152–4.

[38] Lane NE, Bloch DA, Jones HH, Marshall Jr WH, Wood PD, Fries JF. Long-distance running, bone density, and osteoarthritis. JAMA 1986;255(9):1147–51.

[39] Lane NE, Michel B, Bjorkengren A, et al. The risk of osteoarthritis with running and aging: a 5-year longitudinal study. J Rheumatol 1993;20(3):461–8.

[40] Lane NE, Oehlert JW, Bloch DA, Fries JF. The relationship of running to osteoarthritis of the knee and hip and bone mineral density of the lumbar spine: a 9 year longitudinal study. J Rheumatol 1998;25(2):334–41.

[41] Konradsen L, Hansen EM, Sondergaard L. Long distance running and osteoarthrosis. Am J Sports Med 1990;18(4):379–81.

[42] Stenlund B. Shoulder tendinitis and osteoarthrosis of the acromioclavicular joint and their relation to sports. Br J Sports Med 1993;27(2):125–30.

[43] Bollen SR, Wright V. Radiographic changes in the hands of rock climbers. Br J Sports Med 1994;28(3):185–6.

[44] Schmitt H, Hansmann HJ, Brocai DR, Loew M. Long term changes of the throwing arm of former elite javelin throwers. Int J Sports Med 2001;22(4):275–9.

[45] Schmitt H, Brocai DR, Lukoschek M. High prevalence of hip arthrosis in former elite javelin throwers and high jumpers: 41 athletes examined more than 10 years after retirement from competitive sports. Acta Orthop Scand 2004;75(1):34–9.

[46] Roos H, Lindberg H, Gardsell P, Lohmander LS, Wingstrand H. The prevalence of gon-arthrosis and its relation to meniscectomy in former soccer players. Am J Sports Med 1994; 22(2):219–22.

[47] Lindberg H, Roos H, Gardsell P. Prevalence of coxarthrosis in former soccer players. 286 players compared with matched controls. Acta Orthop Scand 1993;64(2):165–7.

[48] Shepard GJ, Banks AJ, Ryan WG. Ex-professional association footballers have an increased prevalence of osteoarthritis of the hip compared with age matched controls despite not having sustained notable hip injuries. Br J Sports Med 2003;37(1):80–1.

[49] Drawer S, Fuller CW. Propensity for osteoarthritis and lower limb joint pain in retired professional soccer players. Br J Sports Med 2001;35(6):402–8.

[50] Turner AP, Barlow JH, Heathcote-Elliott C. Long term health impact of playing professional football in the United Kingdom. Br J Sports Med 2000;34(5):332–6.

[51] Deacon A, Bennell K, Kiss ZS, Crossley K, Brukner P. Osteoarthritis of the knee in retired, elite Australian Rules footballers. Med J Aust 1997;166(4):187–90.

[52] Meir RA, McDonald KN, Russell R. Injury consequences from participation in professional rugby league: a preliminary investigation. Br J Sports Med 1997;31(2):132–4.

[53] Gross P, Marti B. Risk of degenerative ankle joint disease in volleyball players: study of former elite athletes. Int J Sports Med 1999;20(1):58–63.

[54] Hannan MT, Felson DT, Pincus T. Analysis of the discordance between radiographic changes and knee pain in osteoarthritis of the knee. J Rheumatol 2000;27(6):1513–7.

[55] Vertullo CJ, Nunley JA. Participation in sports after arthrodesis of the foot or ankle. Foot Ankle Int 2002;23:625–8.

[56] Hill CL, Gale DG, Chaisson CE, et al. Knee effusions, popliteal cysts, and synovial thickening: association with knee pain in osteoarthritis. J Rheumatol 2001;28(6):1330–7.

[57] Felson DT, McLaughlin S, Goggins J, et al. Bone marrow edema and its relation to progression of knee osteoarthritis. Ann Intern Med 2003;139(5 Pt 1):330–6.

[58] Felson DT, Chaisson CE, Hill CL, et al. The association of bone marrow lesions with pain in knee osteoarthritis. Ann Intern Med 2001;134(7):541–9.

[59] Krampla W, Mayrhofer R, Malcher J, Kristen KH, Urban M, Hruby W. MR imaging of the knee in marathon runners before and after competition. Skeletal Radiol 2001;30(2):72–6.

[60] Maier CF, Tan SG, Hariharan H, Potter HG. T2 quantitation of articular cartilage at 1.5 T. J Magn Reson Imaging 2003;17(3):358–64.

[61] Potter HG, Linklater JM, Allen AA, Hannafin JA, Haas SB. Magnetic resonance imaging of articular cartilage in the knee. An evaluation with use of fast-spin-echo imaging. J Bone Joint Surg Am 1998;80(9):1276–84.

[62] Faber KJ, Dill JR, Amendola A, Thain L, Spouge A, Fowler PJ. Occult osteochondral lesions after anterior cruciate ligament rupture. Six-year magnetic resonance imaging follow-up study. Am J Sports Med 1999;27(4):489–94.

[63] Garnero P, Rousseau JC, Delmas PD. Molecular basis and clinical use of biochemical markers of bone, cartilage, and synovium in joint diseases. Arthritis Rheum 2000;43(5):953–68.

[64] Neidhart M, Muller-Ladner U, Frey W, et al. Increased serum levels of non-collagenous matrix proteins (cartilage oligomeric matrix protein and melanoma inhibitory activity) in marathon runners. Osteoarthritis Cartilage 2000;8(3):222–9.

[65] Lane NE, Bloch DA, Wood PD, Fries JF. Aging, long-distance running, and the development of musculoskeletal disability. A controlled study. Am J Med 1987;82(4):772–80.

[66] Sarna S, Kaprio J, Kujala UM, Koskenvuo M. Health status of former elite athletes. The Finnish experience. Aging (Milano) 1997;9(1–2):35–41.

ELSEVIER
SAUNDERS

Clin Sports Med 24 (2005) 199–203

CLINICS
IN SPORTS
MEDICINE

Index

Note: Page numbers of article titles are in **boldface** type.